Penny O'Connor

Penny O'Connor was training as an actor at Rose Bruford in 1975 when an enlightened voice teacher suggested she take extra classes in a curious thing called Alexander Technique to help her voice. It was a life-changer.

She worked as an actor, playwright, director and teacher until 1992, courtesy of UB40 cards, Arts Council grants, socialist feminist educational theatre companies, such as Half Moon YPT and the Women's Theatre Group, and the Inner London Education Authority.

She qualified as a teacher of the Alexander Technique in 1992 and has been teaching this full-time to fellow thesps and normal people ever since, in London, on the Greek island of Alonnisos, and globally on Zoom. She has taught Alexander at several London drama schools, including ArtsEd, where she was resident for eighteen years, and is currently assisting in training Alexander teachers at the South Bank Alexander Centre.

She is married to the incomparable Mo, loves running, writing and snorkelling in the crystal-clear waters of the Aegean, and recently began mudlarking on the Thames foreshore. She is a member of the Society of Teachers of the Alexander Technique.

www.alexanderpen.co.uk
www.facebook.com/AlexanderTechniqueCityandIslington

Other Movement Books
from Nick Hern Books

THE ARTICULATE BODY
The Physical Training of the Actor
Anne Dennis

BEING A DANCER
Advice from Dancers and Choreographers
Lyndsey Winship

FELDENKRAIS FOR ACTORS
How to Do Less and Discover More
Victoria Worsley

LABAN FOR ACTORS AND DANCERS
Putting Laban's Movement Theory into Practice:
A Step-by-Step Guide
Jean Newlove

LABAN FOR ALL
Jean Newlove and John Dalby

THE SPACE TO MOVE
Essentials of Movement Training
Christian Darley

THROUGH THE BODY
A Practical Guide to Physical Theatre
Dymphna Callery

THE VIEWPOINTS BOOK
A Practical Guide to Viewpoints and Composition
Anne Bogart and Tina Landau

ALEXANDER TECHNIQUE for ACTORS

A Practical Course

Penny O'Connor

Illustrated by Jenny Quick

NICK HERN BOOKS
London
www.nickhernbooks.co.uk

A Nick Hern Book

Alexander Technique for Actors
first published in Great Britain in 2021
by Nick Hern Books Limited,
The Glasshouse, 49a Goldhawk Road, London W12 8QP

Cover image: *8 Minutes* by Alexander Whitley Dance
Company at Sadler's Wells Theatre, London, 2017 (Johan
Persson/ArenaPAL)
Designed and typeset by Nick Hern Books
Printed and bound in Great Britain by
Severn, Gloucester

A CIP catalogue record for this book is available
from the British Library

ISBN 978 1 84842 758 7

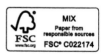

To my sister Christine,
who always loved to hear I was writing a book

Donations to Alzheimer's Research UK gratefully received
www.alzheimersresearchuk.org

When you set out on your way to Ithaca
Pray that your journey be a long one
Full of adventure, full of knowledge.

From 'Ithaca', C. P. Cavafy[1]

Contents

Introduction: Beginners, Please!

The distinguished Alexander teacher Frank Pierce Jones said one should treat every lesson as though it were the first. Both teacher and student need the beginner's mind, the state of unknowing, open to receive, curious and responsive in the moment; working with the actual person present, not the projected memory of who the person was last time we met. It's the state of mind an actor has, who performs a part many times but is fresh each time as though she has never said that line or seen that person before.

When I was first introduced to Alexander Technique, it was a life-changer. The teacher placed one hand on my head and one under my chin and said 'Simply follow your head' as he gently guided me out of a chair in a way I had never experienced before. I arrived at standing without knowing how I had done it. I had no sensation of muscular effort. I was sitting, and then I was standing. It was seamless. I have been trying to work out how that happened ever since. More importantly, I had a deep realisation that there were unknown experiences to be had in this life – that I could be other than I thought I was. And here was someone on my side, who didn't want me to try hard or do something in order to prove something. The teacher allowed me the space to be who I really was and not the pretend Penny that everyone else thought I was. I had crafted Pretend Penny over the years to get by, to protect myself from all the slings and arrows that life had so far thrown at me. As we all do. I was about nineteen. And just by the experience of moving effortlessly for a moment, I had this very powerful inkling that life could be something very different from what I had thought it was. I wondered then if I shouldn't be exploring more of this stuff and forget about the acting lark. I was so moved. But no, I was wanting to be an actor, wasn't I? And, actually, I didn't have a clue how to go about doing more of this stuff! So I stuck to my acting guns.

The Alexander lessons continued – a small group of four of us would visit a training school in West London for our lessons on a Saturday morning – and served me well in my chosen profession. My voice, confidence and transformational acumen, my ability to connect with fellow actors, all developed hugely. I got the lead part in a third-year show! But several years on, I began to run out of steam. I was extremely anxious, impecunious, and my personal life was not easy. At that moment, another Alexander teacher presented herself to me – we do that somehow: we often come along at the right time in someone's life. I treated myself to an individual session, and I knew immediately that I had come home. From then on I organised my life around this desire to learn more and pass on the teachings to others. Once the decision was made, many things conspired to help me: a grant, an opportunity, a space on a training course – it was as if all the traffic lights had turned green.

I feel really blessed to have found this work (or that it found me), and that it has been such a big part of my life. I hope that in some small way this book will bring others to the work, to help them in their acting career and, for some, strike deep to the heart.

How It All Began

Dr Wilfred Barlow, rheumatologist and Alexander's nephew-in-law, described Frederick Matthias Alexander as a showman and a genius, a delightful rogue who had discovered 'a method for making genuine gold bricks.'[1] It started as a means to solve a problem. F. M., as he was known, was an Australian actor who, whilst on tour reciting Shakespeare in the 1880s, began to lose his voice. The doctor diagnosed inflamed vocal cords and irritation of the mucous membrane in his throat and nose, and recommended he rested his voice for two weeks. Alexander's voice came back in time for his next recital, but halfway through the performance the problem returned and by the end he could hardly speak. They agreed that it must be something he was doing to himself. But what? Alexander was determined to find out, proving that we not only need a beginner's mind, open to receive, but also a practical, questing spirit, to find out what habits might be restricting or influencing our performance. His observations took some months, but he eventually realised that, as he started to recite, he pulled his head back, depressing the larynx, and sucked in air through his mouth, which sounded like a gasp. At the same time, he was lifting his chest, thereby arching his back, which shortened his stature and created a pattern of tension throughout his whole body, including the legs. His elocutionist had suggested at one time that he should grip the floor with his feet and this he had faithfully carried out. All this amounted to a very strong pattern that he had cultivated, and he noticed it was something he did, to a lesser extent, even when he was talking normally, not 'on voice'. So that was easy then: once we know which of our habits are causing the problem, we can easily stop them, huh? No? What is the greatest power in the universe? – the power of habit! But Alexander trounced it. He found a way out, and he began teaching his method to others.

Habits are like predictive text on a mobile phone. Alexander found a way of reprogramming his 'predictive text', creating new neural pathways from the brain to the muscle. By stopping and consciously redirecting himself, he found a natural movement and poise that freed the neck, so his head came up, his stature lengthened and widened, his legs released and his throat and breathing were no longer restricted. His voice returned!

Alexander was brought up on and influenced by the Delsarte System, an aesthetic movement very popular in theatre circles at that time that espoused natural movement and gesture influenced by the emotion within – a precursor to the Stanislavsky-based work on which modern acting is founded. Alexander became famous in Australia for his breathing and voice skills, and set up one of the first modern drama schools in Sydney. The Dramatic and Operatic Conservatorium had a syllabus not too dissimilar from what we have today, with lessons in singing, speaking, deportment, gesture and dramatic expression, based on the Delsarte System as well as on Alexander's own work. However, when he moved to London in 1904, he made a clean break from Delsarte's teaching and concentrated on promoting his own method, working with the great actors of the day, including Henry Irving, Viola Tree and Lily Brayton. Writers such as Aldous Huxley and George Bernard Shaw also became devotees. He continued to teach and develop his work internationally, writing four books on the subject, playing Hamlet at the Old Vic, riding, wining, dining and wearing spats to the end of his life in 1955, when he died of influenza. Quite a guy! And his legacy lives on: Alexander Technique is still taught in theatre and music schools throughout the world, as well as to individual acting greats, helping actors perform effortlessly and with confidence, free in their movement and voice.

So the 'Alexander Technique' started as a very practical problem-solving device. But when we start consciously to change a habit, it throws up large questions. What is consciousness? Do we have free will? Are we the sum of our habits or something more than that? If the unconscious has already made a decision before we are aware of it, can we at least disrupt that decision when it does enter our awareness? Am I more than just a jumble of body parts?

Here's what some actors say of his work:

> 'With the best of intentions, the job of acting can become a display of accumulated bad habits, trapped instincts and blocked energies. Working with the Alexander Technique has given me sightings of another way... Mind and body, work and life together. Real imaginative freedom...' Alan Rickman

> '[The Alexander Technique] is a way to transform stress to joy. It's my way of keeping on track with work and truth and the world I'm in, which is working with people and creating.' Juliette Binoche

> 'It's beautiful, an art... it was about being still and relaxed in order to one hundred per cent listen to someone, to be present.' Hugh Jackman

> 'Alexander Technique really helped my posture and focus during my stint as Othello with Northern Broadsides Theatre Company. Imagine how excited I was when I arrived at the National Theatre for *Comedy of Errors* and found I could have Alexander taught to me once a week, I was chuffed to little meatballs.' Lenny Henry

There's an apocryphal story about Michelangelo being asked by a small child what he was doing as he chiselled away at a piece of marble. 'There is an angel trapped in that stone, and I am setting it free,' comes the reply. That is what it felt like to me when my teachers worked with me, allowing me to shed the unnecessary and reveal the essence. That is what I like to think

I am doing when I work with an actor. Together we chip away at the old habits, the old patterns of use, to reveal the Inner Actor. So let's start where it all began, with the practical...

How to Use This Book

We can't read about the Alexander Technique and expect to learn much from it. It will feed your intellectual hunger, perhaps, but if you want to learn to ride a bike, then you have to get on the bike and learn through wobbling about, having someone guiding you, falling off, getting back on, until you magically find your balance – and off you go. So how come I am writing a book for actors on this very subject? There's a paradox somewhere. But I can help you choose a bike and perhaps be the one to have a stabilising hand on your saddle. In this book I hope to get you to experiment for yourself and discover the exhilarating whoosh of freedom Alexander can give you, exploring unknown territory self-propelled, balancing and moving easily as you strut your stuff onstage and on-screen. What follows is a course of eleven lessons based on my years of teaching on the BA and MA theatre courses at the Arts Educational Schools in London, and on my own pathway through the work. I suggest it should take eleven weeks – one week per lesson, including theory, instruction and assignments – but it can be spread over a longer time frame. I have so ordered it that, if all you manage is the first chapter and first assignment, you will leave this book better informed, and will have learned something you can immediately put into practice and add to your actor's toolbox.

As far as possible I have suggested a way for you to experiment on your own: after all, it's your own journey. What you discover may not be what others will discover. It's a personal journey to discover your habits, the way you use yourself in life, and to find a way of relinquishing those that are interfering with your performance. Alexander called his second book *Constructive Conscious Control of the Individual*, and he discovered and developed the work through self-investigation. But you may find it easier to do this in a group or with a study partner, either face to face or online, depending on the circumstances. Read the chapters aloud to each other on Zoom, practise your sight-reading. The art of acting requires other people, either to play off or to support us, to listen and watch us; we are learning to connect, to respond to others, onstage and on-screen. We like working together, we learn more easily and it's fun. In your group or pair for this journey you can encourage each other and give perceptions and insights from an external perspective, understanding your own habits better by witnessing someone else's journey. And if it's not so easy at times, there is someone else's ear to bend, to share and receive inspiration from. Whichever way – online, face to face, on your own, or in a pair/ group – may you have lots of adventures, experience yourself differently, and find ease, lightness, openness, and freedom to choose.

At the start of each lesson you'll find a list of equipment you will need, so best to read ahead to gather what's required. For Lesson Seven, you will need to find a long peacock feather or a light garden cane – you may want to start looking for that peacock feather now! For almost every lesson you will need a long mirror, internet access and filming equipment. This is especially important if you are working on your own: you need to see clearly what you are doing. If you are using your laptop or other device with a platform like Zoom, do make the image as true as possible. You will be aware that the screen will not always show the full head-to-toe image, unless you are some distance from it, and the angle of the screen can give false perspectives. Experiment and use a mirror from time to time too. Your workspace doesn't always have to be large. If you are working at home, you may be able to do some of the major exercises by walking down the hallway or the street or in the park. One or two of the exercises within a chapter you can perhaps read about and assign yourself to do during the week that follows. I suggest you will also need a logbook or blog: stick your first drawing in here and then make notes on your journey. You can go through this course without writing anything down, but writing about your observations and experiments will make for clearer, easier learning.

In Appendix E there is a list of Alexander principles. It may be good to read them at the beginning and feel free to refer to them at any time during the course of your learning if it helps. The principles intertwine within the lessons, so it's not a map, but can be useful as a reference point if you are feeling lost.

The length of time it takes to learn Alexander Technique? The same it takes to learn a musical instrument. It depends, doesn't it? One summer a fifteen-year-old decided to learn the guitar. She took an old instrument and *Bert Weedon's Play in a Day* down to the beach and began to strum. Ouch! Her fingertips took quite a bruising from the steel strings, and it took her more than a day. But she persevered and by the end of the summer could play 'She'll Be Coming 'Round the Mountain' without too many pauses, and in a couple of years was accompanying herself well enough to be singing in folk clubs. That's as far as I wanted to take it. And this was folk, not classical, which is a whole other ball game. So think of this book as a starter. Persevere. It's a solid foundation which can lead you to further, deeper studies and accompany you for the rest of your life.

Lesson One:
The Power of Habit

The nature of habit, discovering our own,
and learning how to let go

Equipment

- A recording device on which to film yourself
- A space big enough to walk up and down in
- A hard-backed chair or stool
- A4 paper
- Coloured pens
- Your logbook/blog
- A delicious snack
- Baroque music
- Headrests or paperback books
- A mat for lying down (optional)

The Nature of Habits

What are habits? How do we acquire them? Can we easily 'experience' ourselves out of them? And what's in it for actors? How can we get out of our habits? What was Alexander's habit?

> 'The brain becomes used to thinking in a certain way, it works in a groove, and when set in action, slides along the familiar, well-worn path; but once it is lifted out of the groove, it is astonishing how easily it may be directed. At first it will have a tendency to return to its old manner of working by means of one mechanical unintelligent operation, but the groove soon fills and although thereafter we may be able to use the old path if we choose, we are no longer bound by it.' F. M. Alexander, *Man's Supreme Inheritance*[1]

Before you read on, and without thinking about it, fold your arms. Now fold them the other way round. How did you get on? Not so easy? Feels weird? What did you have to do to fold them the other way round? I guess you had to think about it, to bring this simple action to consciousness so you could instruct your arms to move differently, and perhaps even then you weren't sure if it was the other way round. Maybe even now it feels 'wrong' and not particularly comfortable. It may bring a smile to your face – it's kind of laughable to be suddenly so incompetent at a relatively easy movement. You are out of your habit. Welcome to the wacky world of Alexander Technique! It's fun, creative and will take you out of your habits so you experience yourself quite differently at times. Be prepared to play. All you had to do was to pause and consciously change how you moved. Our habits are strong and they feel like 'us': we may not want to change actions if we feel we are changing ourselves or our personalities. Relax – we never lose habits entirely. We can always go back to the old ways. They are still there, waiting for us to pick up any time we want. But once we've found a way that lets us move easily, breathe easily, stand easy, sit well, walk tall, why would we want to use effort, holding and fixity?

Experiencing my personal Alexander journey, I find that I have become *more* myself, no longer limited by habit. We only change what we want to change, and it's always our choice. Alexander returns us to self-awareness and conscious choice. We cannot always change the world around us, but we can change our reaction to it. Habits are not necessarily bad things. We are creatures of habit, after all, but we need not be slaves to our habits.

> '... there is nothing either good or bad, but thinking makes it so.' William Shakespeare, *Hamlet*[2]

Alexander is non-judgemental. Habits are habits. Habits are useful. If we didn't retain skills and the knowledge of how to do things unconsciously, we would not be able to develop. But sometimes, when habits are no longer serving us, we may want to change them.

How Did We Get Them?

In her book *My Mother Myself*, Nancy Friday tells a great story.[3] Peggy cooks a huge smoked ham for her parents. Her new husband asks why she cut off the end of the shank before baking it. She looks to her mother. Her mother says that she always did it that way because her mother did it that way too. They phone up the grandma and the reply is the same, 'because her mother did it that way'. Luckily, the great-grandmother is still alive so they call her. The answer is that when Peggy's grandma was little and learning to cook, Great-Grandma only had a small roasting pan and the ham was too big to fit into it, so she cut off the shank end to make it fit. But Peggy doesn't need to do that any more.

Habits start as a good idea at some point. We learn by imitation, taking on our parents' patterns of use. I once saw a delightful, beaming boy thrilled at being on the front seat at the top of a double-decker bus. He was looking around, through thick pebble glasses, sitting up and full of energy and curiosity. Suddenly he sat back and hunched down. It was such a shock, the joy seemed to have been knocked out of him and he looked introspective and sad. What had happened? And then I saw the guy sitting behind him in exactly the same pose – it was clearly his dad. At an early age we model ourselves on our elders. We want to be like our mum and dad.

Another way of acquiring habits is by deliberately cultivating them. Alexander taught himself to grip the floor with his feet as instructed by his elocutionist. If you went to ballet classes as a child you will perhaps stand in turn-out, with a lift to your chest. If soccer was your thing, perhaps you are left with a strong swing action as you walk, and a taut lower back. As we go through adolescence there are so many changes going on, with hormones changing how we think and feel (oh, that time of the month!), our bodies rapidly growing into different shapes and height, the voice becoming squeaky and deeper at the same time. Not surprisingly, our self-consciousness grows and we react to that in different ways, sometimes stooping if we're embarrassed by our height, or trying to hide our breasts. We imitate our friends and heroes rather than our caregivers, sometimes giving up the freedom and ease we had as a child as we try not to stand out from the crowd. Our habits can be defensive, ensuring that we survive. These are not so easy to let go of. But with Alexander you can choose which habits still work for you and which don't. You learn to let go of them, and change how you use yourself. This can feel quite magical, liberating, and challenging.

What's Going On in the Brain?

In Channel 4's *Body Story* series, Episode 7 explains that we are born with only half a brain.[4] Eek! Our brain is an electrochemical system, and the primitive brain is hard-wired, preprogrammed for our survival. We breathe, we grip with our fingers, we cry, we suck, we defecate and we move, albeit chaotically. But the cerebral cortex that governs higher brain functions is not yet fully formed. It is smooth, and the neurons, the brain cells, are not connected. The infant's brain is invaded by outside stimuli, but it cannot immediately make sense of them – we 'see' sound, for example. The connections between the neurons develop quickly in response to our experience of the world. The neurons start wiring themselves together in patterns, so we can make sense of the chaos. The eyes work reflexively, first to recognise faces and then to follow movement. We cry from the word go – it's our first communication and it's a survival mechanism. We need nourishment or we will die: the parent obligingly feeds us.

At about six weeks we smile – purely by accident. But the smile gets us more attention, so we smile again and start communicating beyond the reflexive crying. Adults begin to speak to us in sing-song, which helps the cortex wire itself to be able to distinguish sounds. We are held in our carers' arms and caressed. We begin to distinguish the difference between us and other 'things'. By eight weeks there is so much information coming in from this bizarre world of shape, colour, texture, smell, taste and sound, that we need more brain power to organise it, so the cortex begins to crumple up in order to create more surface area, more space for all the connections. Otherwise there would be no room in our skull! That's when our brains develop that walnut-like appearance.

We develop free will and conscious choice at around ten weeks. The eye reflex that keeps us following whatever moves in front of us is jammed by a signal from the cortex, and we start to turn our head whenever we want to look at something. Over the next four weeks the hand–eye coordination develops through experiment. We now have so many connections we have to start pruning them. When we get close to touching something we want – that squeaky, furry thing with a face on it – those pathways get stronger, and the other pathways, those that fail to get our hand anywhere near our teddy, die off, so that the brain and muscles start working together efficiently. The strongest connections are insulated with glial cells (white matter) to create a stronger and faster signal. And at last the hand goes to where we want it to go – Teddy!

We start to take control of our lives. We create our own programme of neural networks. This pruning and creating new, strong pathways goes on throughout our lives, shaped by our experience. Neuroscience has at last discovered that we go on learning throughout our lives– old dogs can, in fact, learn new tricks and, in the case of Alexander, unlearn old ones. He was ahead of his time. So when you fold your arms in the usual way the strong neural pathway in the brain, insulated with glial cells for a fast, efficient connection, kicks in. The signal from the brain travels down the nerves into the muscles instructing them to contract or release, according to the usual pattern of movement.

The brain, if you like, is the city – lots of interconnecting roads and lanes and streets – and the nerves are the motorways – all made of tarmac. When you fold your arms the other way round, your brain is having to abandon the old pathway and use different ones: it has to fire differently, so your muscles synchronise themselves in a new, orderly fashion. It's not quite as challenging as first learning to move; you can hitch a ride on neural pathways that are already formed and simply shift the order of things. And this is happening because you are consciously choosing to do it, it's no longer an automatic habit. These programmes are not stored in a particular place, it's a whole-brain activity. There are areas such as the sensory and motor cortex, which specialise in receiving and giving signals to the body, but the amygdala – the emotional centre of our brain – is also connected to movement. Perhaps you learned to cross your arms as a defence when an elder was telling you off about some misdemeanour, or when you were bored and not wanting to be there. And as we move, the cerebellum at the back of the brain also seems to be monitoring how we perform a movement, reminding us of our habit if we are moving differently.

Why Do Actors Need to Know About Their Habits?

If you are using too much tension, pulling down, collapsing or bracing yourself to hold yourself up, you will not perform so well. Your voice may be affected, you may not be heard, you may not be able to breathe well, or take on the physicality of a character. You may even be injuring yourself – stressing the discs in your spine, for example, or inflaming your vocal cords. To borrow a motoring analogy, if we use a car badly by driving with the handbrake on, it won't function very well. It won't go very fast, it will be using up too much petrol and it will wear out the brake linings. Alexander teachers are like driving instructors. We teach you to take the handbrake off, to come out of your habits and reorganise your neural pathways so you can use yourself well.

It is also important for transformation. As an actor you inhabit someone else's world, you explore someone else's thoughts and patterns of behaviour, their habits of speech and movement as revealed through the text, explored in rehearsal and interpreted by you and the director. You create the neural network of another character in your own brain. You don't want to bring your own habits along, unless it's appropriate to the character. So if you want to play someone else, it's good to understand something of yourself first in order to discern what you need to lose and what you can keep. You may need to change your accent, your shape, your movement pattern. Sir

Laurence Olivier was famous for wanting to transform himself entirely, using all sorts of make-up and false noses in order to change his outward appearance, as well as finding the truth of the character from within. Late in his career he was asked in an interview why, in view of this, he continued to lick his lips in a particular way whatever role he was playing. He was aghast! He didn't know he'd been doing this. Our habits can be writ large onstage and on-screen, so best get to know your own. Learn to inhibit them and inhabit instead a neutral or centred place as your starting point, a creative space in which your ego/habits are jettisoned so you can respond in the moment and ensure your potential to become something other than you thought you were.

You not only need to inhabit the unknown but also to feel comfortable with it. This is the quality of the creative space where we can play and have adventures. Try this one:

Drawing Yourself

After you've read these instructions, put some music on – preferably baroque, such as Bach, Handel or Vivaldi – and treat yourself to a nice snack. As you are relishing it, take a piece of A4 paper and some coloured pens and, with your non-dominant hand, draw a picture of yourself. Write your name on it, also with your non-dominant hand. (If you are ambidextrous, use both hands at the same time.) Halfway through, stop drawing but freeze in that position. What do you notice? Are you tensing yourself unnecessarily? What are you leaning on? How is your back? Feel free to change any of this as you become aware and continue your drawing. In that moment you are embodying Alexander, becoming aware of how you are doing something, pausing and choosing to change it – directing yourself.

Now turn the paper over and write with your usual hand. Enjoy feeling skilled again whilst perhaps being slightly more conscious of how you are doing this. Write down five habits of movement, speech and balance you know you have. For example, I always walk fast; I often cross my legs when I sit; I usually lean back in a chair; I walk with a swagger. Keep this paper – you'll be adding to it later.

This is not an exercise in how well you draw, but an exercise in what it feels like to be incompetent and out of your usual habit. Did you find yourself smiling, having a laugh? 'The work is too serious to be taken seriously!'[5] Alexander is rumoured to have said. When we are serious we tend to stiffen up, frown, concentrate – another enormous habit, and very trying. It's good practice to be open, light, playful, experimenting. I hope you enjoyed the snack and the music. The snack was to feed the kinaesthetic sense, the music the auditory sense. Did you know baroque music orders the brain, so it calms down and learns more easily?[6] If you are working in a pair/group, by all means enjoy looking at each other's drawings – you'd be surprised how uncannily accurate they can be.

Raising Your Hand

Raise your right arm in the air, then take it down to your side again. How did you do that? Where did the movement start? Did it start with the muscles of the shoulder, the upper arm? Did your shoulder lead or your hand? Is it the same with your other arm? If it was your shoulder that led the movement, raise the arm again but this time let the hand lead, as if there were a string attached to the back of your hand like a marionette... and down again. How was that? If it was your hand that led, see how it feels when you let your shoulder lead the movement, and don't bend the elbow. Feel the difference? Which way do you prefer? (That last way of moving the arm reminds me of school: 'Please, Miss, I know the answer!' or 'Please, Miss, I need to go to the loo!') Repeat this experiment with the left arm – do you move it in the same way? Is it easier to change?

Think again of raising your right arm. But only think it. Our habits are there before we take action. Our brain has decided that we are about to move and will bring out the old programme we developed as kids. It's the predictive-text thing I mentioned earlier. You may sense this as you think of moving the right arm. It's as though the arm has filled up with thought in preparation to move. In this instance we want to inhibit the neural pathway from brain to muscle in the top of the arm or shoulder, and instead ask the hand to lead. Now let it move, hand leading.

From now on, every time you go to move your arm you can pause and choose which way you do it. I suggest that allowing the hand to lead will be a more graceful, effortless movement and may be the one you want to start practising if it's not your usual way. But it's your journey and your choice.

We don't just have personal habits, we have sociocultural ones too, ranging from the clothes we wear to our attitudes to money or morality. One of these is continuing to view the mind and body separately, despite the popular holistic movement of alternative medicine. As actors, we know we are interconnected, psycho-physical beings. Alexander rarely referred to the body but used the words 'mechanism' or 'self' or 'organism'. Our feelings and thoughts are manifested in our physicality. Our physicality can also affect our thoughts. Let me ask you to take a couple of minutes to imagine that the right side of your face is covered in greenish scabby scales... I suspect that you have already begun to change how you are reading this, how you are sitting, and perhaps already a small story has arisen as to how and when your scales got there and some emotional response is kicking in. Perhaps you try to hide the face, perhaps you display it happily or defiantly to the world. This is what your audience will read. It needs no words. How many actual words do you remember from a play or film? Maybe some famous ones like 'To be or not to be' or 'Tomorrow is another day'.

But what we remember most clearly are the visuals, the emotions and the story. And the consummate skill of the actor who conveys all this. So bear this in mind: in the Alexander Technique we are not addressing just postural habits, but how we are manifesting our thoughts and emotions through our whole selves.

Luckily, the brain loves doing things differently. It enjoys learning – remember how you smiled when you folded your arms the wrong way round or drew the picture with your non-dominant hand? Another sociocultural habit is how we learn. Often we are educated to try hard to get things right, to pass the tests, to please others, to hurry up, be strong, be perfect. You can stop all that with Alexander Technique. How would it be if we allowed ourselves to get things wrong, to play, to not take tests, to be imperfect, to please ourselves, to learn at a pace that suits us, to be flexible, to create more with less? What a wonderful world that would be! In order to learn we need to make mistakes. Apparently, the guy who invented Post-it notes was trying to make a better superglue. Nice one! No experiment ever 'fails': it gives us information and, in that sense, succeeds every time. 'Trying is only emphasising the thing we know already,' as Alexander said.[7] Learning takes the time it takes. He never used the phrase 'the Alexander Technique', he called it 'the Work'. But I generally invite people not to work at it, but to play with it, experiment, discover.

Let's take up Alexander's story for a moment. In many ways his attitude was very pragmatic. As we have seen, the Technique started in the world of theatre as a solution to a voice problem. Passionate about theatre, poetry, Shakespeare and reciting, Alexander had dedicated himself to becoming professional. Imagine his dismay, then, when he heard himself becoming hoarse and gasping for air. If acting is the love of your life and your voice packs up and you get no help from the medics, what would you do? Give up? Or find a way to help yourself? Fortunately for us, Alexander chose the latter, observing himself in a mirror to work out what habitual actions might be causing the problem.

So, if you want to follow the Alexander Technique, not only will you have to learn to enjoy being in the unfamiliar space of being 'out of habit', you will need to feel comfortable in observing yourself in a mirror, and/or filming yourself and watching the playback. These days we are all quite used to greeting our lovely mugs on Zoom, so I'm sure all will be well. I am quite sure that F. M. would have used Zoom, film, a smartphone, an iPad, whatever he could get his hands on, to discover what it was he was doing. But in the nineteenth century, he only had mirrors. We cannot change our habits using what it feels like from within, because our feelings are not always accurate. If I ask you to stand upright, you may feel you're standing straight but when you look at yourself in profile in the mirror you might see yourself leaning backwards. And when you use the mirror to correct that, you might feel yourself to be leaning forward or hunching, despite the reflection showing you to be upright. You need to change the habit of relying on your feelings. They are accurate in as much as they have registered change – you are further forward than you were – but the interpretation of the change is faulty. Alexander called this 'Faulty Sensory Appreciation'. Our system has adapted to our funny ways, so our habitual way of standing feels normal.

We may have an unreliable body map, too. Let me ask you – where are your hip joints? Where does your head meet your neck? Exactly where are your shoulders? Where does your arm begin and end? What shape are your sitting bones? Where is your diaphragm? How do you know that? And if you asked someone else, they may well answer differently. We also need to look at our habitual beliefs about our movement patterns, because what we believe can dictate how we move. If I think my head turns from the bottom of my neck, then that is how I will do it. Yet we are designed to turn the head at the *top* of the neck. Ah-ha! A person's habit of dropping their neck may be corrected simply by changing their belief as to where the head turns.

To sum up, the Alexander Technique helps us become aware of our habits and gives us a way of letting go of them if they are limiting or restricting our performance. We can then transform effortlessly, speak clearly, move well in any shape we need for our character, receive and act on direction, and be electrifying onstage and on-screen. We'll be embodying great presence, becoming vulnerable, sexy, unpredictable and intelligent, the four qualities a great actor needs. Sound good? Then let's start. Find out what your habits are and how you use yourself through some very simple activities.

Filming Yourself

Find a space to film yourself and set up your device or film equipment so that you can be seen head-to-toe, not just head and shoulders. You're going to be moving and you want to be able to see the whole of yourself easily. You want the image to be as true as you can make it, so have your device at the right height and the screen at right angles, not sloping back or forward. Place a chair halfway in the space sideways to camera, so you can be seen in profile when sitting. If you are doing this with a study partner in a live space, take it in turns to film each other. In a live study group, take it in turns, have someone else film you, and you can have your ready-made audience sitting in front of you.

Next, choose some text from a piece you know well – just a line or two, not a whole speech – and a line or two from a song. Doesn't matter if you think you can't sing, do it anyway; it will give you information. Stand facing camera in full shot and say: 'Hi, my name is... and I am going to speak a line of text from... and sing a line of song from...' Then stand in front of the chair and sit and stand twice in profile, turn away from the camera and walk away to the back of the room. Walk back towards the chair and turn again in profile, as you were standing before. Pick up something imaginary from the floor and place it on an imaginary high shelf. Then speak your line of text and sing your line of song, staying in profile to the camera. Film over. Now look back at it several times and analyse what you are doing. Find the drawing you did of yourself with your non-dominant hand with the list of five of your habits on the back. Are they present in the film? I also want you to look specifically for these:

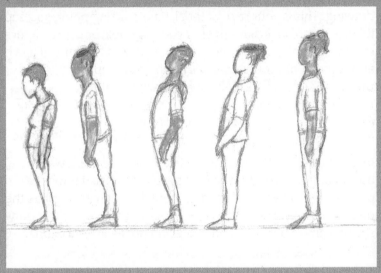

Are you standing upright? Are you leaning forward or backwards? Are your knees locked? Do they come towards each other as you sit?

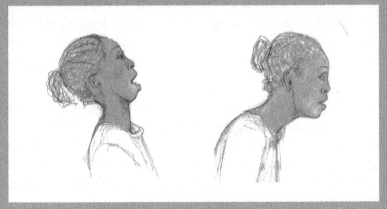

Do you look down a lot? Does your face rise up, tipping the head back as you stand and sit? Does it rise up, tipping the head back to speak or sing? Do your head and neck poke forward all the time, or perhaps only when you speak or sing? Do you have an aura of ease or are you excited, nervous, self-conscious? If you have a study companion, what have they noticed about you?

Write down everything you have noticed on the back of the drawing. This is your raw material, your starting point, so keep it. Stick it into the inside cover of your logbook, or take a picture of it for your blog. And keep the film. You will film yourself again at the end of the course and will be able to compare the two, giving you excellent feedback as to how far you've changed. If you look at the 'Before and After' films on my YouTube channel (youtube.com/ pennyoconnor1) you will see examples of this.

In some of those theatre students the development was huge, but do bear in mind that this was after thirty-six lessons taken over nearly two years of acting school. Sometimes it will be the quality of movement that has changed, sometimes the body shape, sometimes the confidence and presence you exude.

Time Out

Time for a rest and a recap. So far I've been getting you to discover a little more about habits – physical, mental, emotional, sociocultural – and how they are formed. We have examined Alexander's own habits, and why it's useful for an actor to recognise and let go of theirs, experiencing themselves 'out of habit'.

Enough for one lesson, surely? Yes, but I want to finish this week's session by setting up an assignment that will be ongoing and start you immediately on the path to letting go of unwanted habits. Welcome to the art of lying down in semi-supine: 'Constructive Rest' or, as it is sometimes known, 'The Balanced Resting State'.

'Which book changed my life? The one the teacher put under my head during the Alexander Technique sessions at RADA. I grew an inch and a half.' Jonathan Pryce[8]

The Balanced Resting State

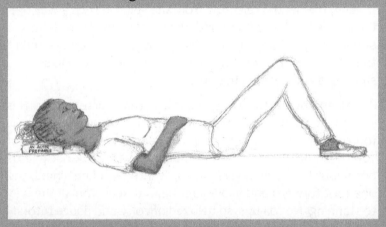

Read the following instructions first and then have a go.

Lie on the floor on your back in semi-supine position – knees up, feet flat on the floor, your head supported by a book or two, or by firm foam headrests. You need it to be just enough support so that your head is not falling back, and not so much that your head restricts your throat. This will give you a healthy alignment between the head, neck and back. Your eyes remain open but resting; not glazing over, not straining. Your hands can rest at your side, palm up or palm down as suits you best. Or they can lie on your belly, palm down.

At the outset, have a wriggle to ensure no clothing is digging in. You may also find it helpful to first do a spinal roll on the floor. Take the head support away. Using your feet for support, and not squeezing your buttocks or abdominals, let the pelvis and spine peel off the floor slowly until you reach the base of your neck, and then roll the spine gently back down again, lowering the pelvis back onto the floor. This will sometimes lengthen and realign the spine. With a hand under your head, lift it and place it back on the headrests. Then leave yourself alone. 'Scan' your body with your mind and be aware of how much of you is on the floor. Remain lying in this position, eyes open, for ten to twenty minutes. As you lie there – without your having to do it, and whether you are aware of it or not – the neck is freeing, the head is releasing from the spine in such a way that the whole back lengthens and widens, and the limbs let go of unnecessary holding and tension, whilst being reconnected to the whole of you. (NB. When I use the word 'back' I include the shoulders and pelvis in this area.)

At the end of ten to twenty minutes, scan yourself again. Has something changed? Come to standing by rolling over onto all fours, being careful not to drop the neck but letting the top of your head be directed to the opposing wall. Rock backwards onto your heels, then rock upwards into high kneeling; bring one foot forward and allow your head to lead you all the way to standing. No roll-ups, so beloved of voice and dance tutors! I want you to maintain the alignment of the head, neck and back that you have just given yourself.

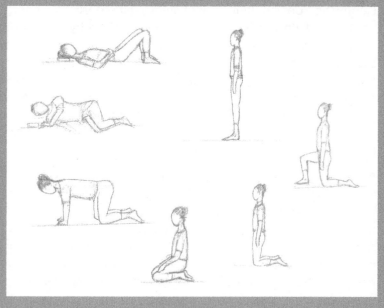

Pause there in standing, and check out how you feel before returning to the book. Okay, having read these instructions, now carry them out.

As you stood there, how did you feel? Lighter, heavier, taller, nearer the ground, floaty, more wobbly, relaxed, energised? About the same? Whatever you experience is entirely valid. There is no right way to do this. It's *your* journey and your experience. What happened as you lay down? Maybe you felt rested, or perhaps your mind was churning with a problem you brought with you to the floor. Maybe you noticed that some pains and discomforts had gone away. Or you may have found it difficult to stay awake. We never step in the same river twice. So each time will be similar and sometimes very different.

Camilla Cleese recently tweeted, 'My dad is the only person on the planet still using a phone book...' – with a picture of John Cleese, a long-term devotee of the Alexander Technique, lying in semi-supine with his head resting on an old copy of *Yellow Pages*.

Doing this as a daily practice will change your life. If you don't do it already, then of course it will be a change! It is a change for many people simply to lie there and not be busy getting on with something more important. This is *very* important. You are learning to quieten yourself, to pay attention and gently experience yourself as a psycho-physical being. At the same time you are letting go of your habits of mind and body, finding that relaxed alertness or alert relaxation, the default you need as an actor. I suggest you do this for ten to twenty minutes every day during your journey through this book. It's an essential ongoing assignment. Keep a record of your daily experience over these eleven weeks in your logbook or blog. It's quite fun to have a note of your discoveries and experiences to look back on. But you will learn anyway, despite yourself. We are naturally learning creatures; it's what happens, we are primed for it.

We don't have to 'do' learning, we learn through our experience. We gain knowledge and wisdom through living. Just turning up regularly and lying down will alter something. And if you write something about it, or draw a picture of it immediately afterwards, it helps the brain retain the experience.

Here are some experiences from drama students who were asked to lie down for twenty minutes every day during one Christmas break:

> 'When I decided to lie down in semi-supine and run lines I actually found that I remembered a lot more.'

> 'Noticed that my exhale is always so shaky. Particularly round my diaphragm area. I feel this has come from holding grief in this area and consequently not breathing properly.'

> 'When I get up and look in the mirror I look taller and more in control of myself. It makes me think of some British actors that have a similar posture, Tom Hardy or Dominic Cooper. That's what this posture looks like. Maybe they've had Alexander Technique training too? I walk round the flat feeling quite cocky with that Tom Hardy/Dominic Cooper air.'

> 'I was working over the holidays as Santa Claus at Heathrow Airport. I would lie down in semi-supine for ten minutes during my hour lunchbreak and when I got home in the evening. Which made wearing an itchy beard and a big belly, and generally being jolly for nine hours on my feet, much more bearable.'

> 'After only lying a minute I felt an extraordinary sensation of relief as my muscles and joints began to soften into the floor and gradually give up the enormous amount of tension they had evidently been holding. As they blissfully surrendered to the floor it became apparent to me that my body had been fairly cramped and trapped for a long time.'

Let's go back to the folding of the arms. First fold them the usual way, then the new way. Repeat several times. Perhaps this is already beginning to feel more familiar? If you continue to repeat these movements, you soon won't even have to think about it – you will have created a new neural pathway from brain to muscle, a new habit, something you can do automatically. Our brains can learn fast. As Alexander said, 'We can throw away the habit of a lifetime in a few minutes if we use our brains.'[9]

The key is remembering to do this – and therein lies the rub. More of this in Lesson Two.

Assignments

- Become aware of your habits as you go through your life this week. Become aware but don't try to change them yet. Exercise non-judgement. Practise observing yourself in a full-length mirror, or in shop windows, so that you can be objective.

- Lie down in semi-supine every day as described above and record your findings in the logbook. How do you feel; what happens to you during and after the event?

- Read through the principles of Alexander Technique in Appendix E.

Have a good week lying down. More fun and games next week!

Lesson Two:
It's the Thought
That Counts

*Experimenting with different ways
of thinking*

Equipment

- A3 or A4 paper
- Coloured pens
- A chair
- A table
- Space to run
- Your logbook

'What distinguishes the Alexander Technique from all other methods of self-improvement that I know anything about is the character of thinking involved… To me it is an expansion of the field of consciousness (or of "attention" if you object to the term "consciousness") in space and time so that you are taking in both yourself and the environment, both the present moment and the next. It is a unified field organised round the self as centre… You can take in what you are doing now and what you are going to do next without getting tangled up on the process… The expanded field of consciousness makes possible what Dewey called "thinking in activity".' Frank Pierce Jones[1]

In this week's lesson we will reflect on how your journey is going, explore habits of mind-wandering, concentration and end-gaining, and find ways of paying attention effortlessly to bring you to consciousness and give you greater presence onstage. Alexander Technique is one of conscious control, so you need to hone your skills of consciousness. If you want to discern and change your habits consciously, you need to learn to be present, to have a unified field of attention that takes in the world around you. You can then respond appropriately to the stimulus you are receiving.

How did your assignments go? Are you getting used to observing yourself and discovering your habitual ways? Have a few moments of reflection on this; look through your log or share your experiences with your study group or partner. Bringing awareness to the way you are doing something whilst you are doing it is not always easy but it is already beginning the journey to widening your attention, as advanced by Frank Pierce Jones above. Bringing to consciousness the way you are doing something is essential if you wish to change it. However, here's the interesting thing: in the simple act of widening your attention you have already changed your behaviour. Mostly our habits are unconsidered; they're to do with some learned reaction from the past. Bringing them to present consciousness gives us the opportunity to change them or to allow change to occur. As we become present, the physical manifestation of habit will already begin to shift. If you are not sure what I mean, this will become clearer by the end of this lesson, so hang on in there!

Paying Attention

Let's go back to the semi-supine experiment. Was it easy to manage? Check out your logbook or feel free to discuss again in your study group or pair.

> 'You'd think an imperative to lie down for twenty minutes every day could be easily followed. Oh, how I wish that I could explain why this isn't so.' Greg, MA acting student

Some people like to find a suitable time and stick to it, timetabling it into their day. At one time I found first thing in the morning best, whilst I was waiting for the coffee to brew. It set me up for the day. I once suggested this to a group of musical-theatre students, as a group experiment for a week. Result: whilst some enjoyed it, a lot disliked having to get up earlier, or they fell asleep again, or were constantly worrying about not getting to college on time. Conclusion? Find the time that works best for you.

If you find your legs won't stay up in the knees-raised position without clenching, place a blanket or similar over the knees. This will stop the legs falling apart but allow the hips to let go. After some weeks of practice the length of muscle in the legs will change and you will have learned to balance them effortlessly. If your lower back is very arched and the sacrum at the bottom of your spine becomes sore, place a folded scarf under the sacrum. It will be more comfortable, and by raising the pelvis it will release the lower back muscles and, over several weeks, undo the overly arched lumbar spine. This will take time and cannot be rushed. If you find it hard to keep your eyes open and want to fall asleep, don't worry. At present your brain is associating lying down with sleep. Or maybe you are simply very tired and need to sleep, and without habitual distractions it's letting you do what you need to do. Zzz... This will pass! Meantime, keep your eyes open as much as possible. We want your brain to associate relaxed alertness with daily activities, and this won't work if you can only find that easy alert state by closing your eyes. Sometimes, however, we deliberately close our eyes so we can 'see' our inner world better, to help us 'concentrate'. Please don't do this. This is a habit of thinking that we want you to avoid in Alexander Technique. ('What? I've spent all these years following the instructions of my teachers and parents to concentrate hard and you are telling me *not* to do this?' Yes, I'm afraid so. Let me put it this way: you're already good at doing that, so you don't need to practise it any more. This other way of thinking will extend your repertoire.)

> 'I do not believe in any concentration that calls for effort. It is the wish, the conscious desire to do a thing or think a thing which results in adequate performance.'
> F. M. Alexander[2]

Just for a moment, concentrate on something, or ask your partner to concentrate on something – a place, an object, a person. What is happening, what change goes on?

Perhaps you noticed the breath getting shallow or even stopping, the eyes closed or screwed up, a frown on the face, the muscles in the shoulders tightening? It's a very common practice. Did your teachers ever tell you to sit up and concentrate? Mine did, and I distinctly remember in my primary school everybody sitting cross-legged on the floor, pushing their chests up and raising their shoulders, staring hard at the teacher so she would think we were concentrating and give us a gold star for being good. So, as we use our screens, mobiles, laptops, tablets, desktops, etc., do we not also narrow our focus and over-tighten our muscles as we concentrate on the work or game or conversation we are having? And the real world around us disappears. Perhaps some of you are concentrating hard to take in this section of the book. We have been groomed to think that this is the way learning happens. Well, I'm not watching and I don't care how you look as you listen or read. So give all that up, let go of any unnecessary holding patterns so you can read and listen effortlessly. Pay attention, yes, but no need to concentrate.

'But if I don't concentrate my mind gets distracted and wanders off!' This is the second habit of thinking that we want to avoid in Alexander Technique. Did any of you find last week that you noticed the antics of your mind more than your body? That as you lay there for your twenty minutes, your mind wandered off to think about what you were about to do, what you had done, wondering how soon you could get up and start being busy again? Or perhaps you started thinking about your cat snuggling up by your neck and purring loudly, and ended up thinking about how that green shirt you saw in the little pop-up shop in Old Street would look perfect for the audition for *Robin Hood* next week, and 'I wonder how Lucy is getting on at Nottingham Uni this term and perhaps she will come with me when I visit Great Uncle Michael in Cornwall. I liked that film *Withnail and I*. Is it the time of year for daffodils...?'

Oh yes, we all have those trains of thought that chug along unhindered. The mind is constantly chattering to itself. Our habit very often is to get caught up in this bubbling dream-like stream of thoughts, paying attention to it instead of paying attention to the outside world and the present moment. There are many meditation disciplines to help us avoid getting caught up in this jumble. One of my first Alexander teachers, who was also a Buddhist nun, suggested that I think of a blue sky with clouds of thought travelling across it and instead of plunging into the cloud of thought, I could stay back and watch the clouds pass by. This image has helped me a lot over the years.

Apparently our clouds of thought are very repetitive. Most of the time we are not having new thoughts, but going over old stuff and old plans again and again. But what is happening to the rest of us as we let the mind do its own thing? Our body is often in a holding pattern, on automatic pilot, offline, in our own world, in our habits. We can tell when someone else is not present; their eyes go 'dead'. Actually, their eyes have stopped moving. When we are truly present and alive, our eyes sparkle. They are moving gently all the time, refracting the light as we take in the visual world, clearly demonstrable when we are back online and able to respond.

Both mind-wandering and concentration are things we need to avoid as actors. Great actors need to be responsive, to have oceans of attention, to be here now and gain that delightful quality of presence onstage. So as a start, practise keeping your eyes open in semi-supine. You will not know when you have wandered off; you'll only be conscious of it when you come back. So, congratulate yourself for coming back when you do. No 'Oh damn, I did it again' wallowing in self-pity whilst slapping your wrist. It's part of the human condition, and people spend a lifetime exploring this hinterland of thinking. This is only your second lesson in the wonders of Alexander Technique.

I was a very good mind-wanderer. It was either that or concentrating to the point of nausea and acute anxiety. Staying gently present was not easy at all. I had to learn to pay attention differently. It's all very well saying, 'Be here now!' but that's like teaching juggling by saying 'Throw the balls up in the air, one after the other and catch them!' I needed some small steps to practise. So here's something I devised to help myself. We can't stop the mind chattering, it's a fundamental condition of being human, but maybe we can occupy it with chatter about what we are actually doing. I am no longer paying attention to a stream of random thoughts but to what I am experiencing now in the outside world. That way the mind and body are involved in the same thing, experiencing a psycho-physical unity.

Cataloguing: Training the Mind to Stay Present

Using Your Visual Attention

As you sit there or walk about the room, talk aloud for a minute or two, naming what you can see. If you are working in a pair or a group you can all do this at the same time; no one else needs to hear what you are saying and you can repeat as much as you like if you find yourself running out of things to see. But my bet is you won't. If you say you see a wall, next time you look at it you might notice the marks on the wall. Be as detailed as you like but leave out any value judgement of what you see. Rather than seeing a 'nice' hat, see a 'battered green' hat: it's simply what it is. Be careful, too, not to add a story to it: 'I see a battered green hat I wore to the theatre last night and would have lost on the Tube in the closing doors if that gorgeous man hadn't grabbed it for me, I was so embarrassed…' It may be that a story flashes through your mind, but this is excellent practice in cutting off the story and simply describing what you see. You are cataloguing, not storytelling. Move on. 'I see a battered green hat, I see a window with a piece of coloured glass. I see a rug, multicoloured, on the floor. I see the laptop I am typing this up on. I see a sculpture to my left, I see my papers on the desk, I see an old motorbike helmet, I see a violin by the fireplace…' Off you go, don't wait for me to stop! 'I see…'

How did you get on? Were you thinking about anything else as you catalogued what you could see? My guess is no. As we allow our attention to embrace the outside world, we are no longer distracted by the inner thoughts or judgements, we are wholeheartedly just doing this simple task. Now try this one:

Using Your Auditory Attention

Catalogue everything you can hear and tune in to where it's coming from. This time talk silently to yourself, as otherwise you will just hear your own or others' voices. Talk to yourself about what you can hear.

It's not that the sounds weren't there before, we just didn't pay them conscious attention. Not so many sounds to distinguish as visual stimuli? Well, human beings are very visually orientated. But, again, I guess that you were more present, more attentive, as your whole brain paid attention to receiving sounds. Now this:

Using Your Kinaesthetic and Olfactory Attention

Let's go back to speaking aloud, and this time talk about what you can sense of the outside world. What is in touch with you? What is the temperature, the feeling of the floor under your feet? Include fragrances, too. If you run out of new sensations, just keep repeating.

Again, there are not so many words for what we feel, or smell. We don't have the refinement to distinguish the differences. If a dog were able to communicate in words, he would have a huge vocabulary for smell!

Using Your Motor Attention

Talk through your actions. For example, as I write this I can write down what I am doing now: 'I am typing into my laptop and I am making contact with the keys on my laptop and I am looking at the screen and sitting with my legs crossed and holding my arms up a little from the keyboard and I'm leaning back in the chair and having a wider vision of the space I am in and letting my arms and shoulders release. I am resting my wrists on the laptop and I am looking through a pair of glasses. I am key-stroking, I am key-stroking, and I am correcting my typos...' I immediately became more aware of my actions in typing this page and changed how I was using myself. And it was very easy. I became present, I wasn't just narrowed to the words and the meaning but to how I was doing it.

Now your turn, and to make it more interesting, let me ask you to move about the room and randomly pick things up and put them down somewhere else. As you do this, talk through what you are doing out loud. Avoid the expression 'going to', as in 'I am going to put the book on the table', which is a future thought. Instead, use the present continuous – 'I am walking, I am putting the book on the table, I am turning and walking towards the sofa, I am walking, I am walking, I am picking up a cushion from the sofa.' Keep repeating what you are doing until you change what you are doing. Off you go. Don't read any more, try it out and then come back.

Result? Thinking presently. Not planning, but coming to a state of improvisation and creativity. Taking action in a non-doing way. Not doing but responding to things you see and deciding to move. Not 'I've got to do this to be entertaining or interesting', just things happening that you hadn't anticipated, because you chose in the moment to move something from one place to the other. If this was a group or pair activity you may have started interacting with each other. It has been known during this exercise that weird artworks have been created with shoes and chairs and bags, that balls are thrown and water bottles snatched, and this all happens effortlessly, not by trying hard or concentrating but simply paying attention to the here and now. If you're familiar with Meisner's teaching, this may remind you of his repetition exercise. I invented it before I read anything of Meisner, but how pleasing to note that we both understood in our separate ways how a repetition in the end brings us to a present, truthful responsiveness.[3]

So there we have 'cataloguing' exercises that might help you to stop the mind-wandering.

The World Changes As We Change Our Attention

Looking for Blue and the New

Have a look around you. What do you see? After the last exercises you are probably very familiar with the room you are in. Stop reading for a moment and take notice of everything blue in the room. Without doing anything, your brain has now highlighted that colour and you will see blue things. The landscape of the room hasn't changed, the blue things were always there, but your perception has changed. I am leading your perceptions, whereas before you perceived the room through your own filter, the way you habitually look at the room.

Stop reading again for a moment and look round for five things you hadn't noticed before. Now your attention will be one of actively searching. I bet you found at least one thing you hadn't consciously noticed before, even if you didn't get to five.

Receiving the world and actively seeking are different ways of paying attention. And we have habits around that. Frank Pierce Jones suggests what we need is a unified field of attention. I sometimes call it a SEA of consciousness – Self, Environment and Activity. We need an even mix of attention between all these three. Too often we cherry-pick or narrow our attention to one of these spheres, and most often it is our activity. We concentrate so hard on what we are doing and our goals, we forget about how we are doing it with no sense of ourselves and with little notion of what is around us. However, if we continue in that vein, our system will let us know with what Pierce Jones describes as a 'nagging discomfort'.

Paying Attention to the Self

In the early twentieth century, coal-miners would bring canaries into the mine as an early-warning system: if the canary fell unconscious it was an indication that there was toxic gas in the mine and the miners needed to get the hell out.

Often we are not aware of ourselves at all – until something hurts. When part of us aches, our attention immediately goes to that part. The pain brings us back to the present moment and we will stop what we are doing. It is often indicating that we were in a narrowed concentrated state, using excessive tension and unnecessary muscular effort. And we take action to soothe it by massaging it directly or moving it around a little. This may help temporarily but weirdly the discomfort often comes back, sometimes worse than before. What we need to do is not revive the canary, but get out of the mine. We can do this by widening our attention.

Here's a plan: if your shoulder is 'killing you', extend your attention to take in the whole arm. The shoulder is still there but is now part of the upper limb. Include the other shoulder and arm into your field of attention, then your neck, your head, the whole of your torso, your legs. The shoulder is still there but now it's in a wider landscape of your whole self. Continue to widen the attention to take in the surrounding environment. I am not suggesting you ignore the shoulder – after all, it's the early-warning system that something's not right – but just to respond differently, to include the shoulder in a wider awareness. As your awareness grows, your shape will subtly change, the muscles release. And that pain may become less acute or even go. If it was caused by how you were sitting, you will have changed that. This widening of your attention so not to get fixed on one part of you is crucial to Alexander's teaching. It's good to practise this whether you have pain or not.

From the Part to the Whole

Right now, think of a part, any part – the tummy, the throat, your big toe – and begin widening your attention to the area around the part. Let the area of awareness increase to take in more and more of you until you are able to take in your whole self as well as the room you are inhabiting, the space around you. It is a simple exercise, but very powerful. It may take time for the narrowed thinking habits to let go and for you to experience the whole self in this way. But keep at it.

Make a fist and release one finger. Take hold of that finger with the other hand and try to move it. How released is it? Now release the whole fist and test the finger again – it will be much more released. We work best as a psycho-physical whole, in relationship to the world outside of ourselves.

To help his voice, Alexander would pay attention to his neck, his head, his back and his legs, one after the other, *all at the same time*. He recognised that a narrowed attention would not help.

Attention to Our Movement

Put a sheet of paper on the table in front of you – A3 is good but A4 would do. Have a coloured felt tip in easy reach. Now forget about those props and gently move your dominant hand forward and back, up and down and around in circles in the air in front of you. Remember how in the last chapter I was getting you to use the arm with the hand leading? Let the hand lead as you explore the movement of your arm – big circles, small circles; let the wrist rotate one way and the other; turn the thumb over the little finger to rotate the lower arm, and back. The focus is on the abstract movement of the arm moving through space. Now take the felt tip in your hand and continue the abstract movements. Can you involve the pen without it meaning anything other than just an extension of your arm?

Now check where the paper is on the table, then close your eyes and allow the pen to make contact with the paper as your arm continues to move in an abstract way. Now open your eyes and continue to move the arm in that abstract way as you watch the marks appear on the paper.

What happened to your attention then? Were you able to keep a sense of the abstract movement of the arm or did you get involved in drawing patterns on the paper, your brain leading the movement to create something specific? Did your attention get drawn and narrowed to the paper and pen, and did the sense of your arm and the space around get lost a little or altogether?

I remember once working with a group of dancers. They were in deep *plié* and I asked them to move their arms up and down three times and then, when their arms hung down the last time, to swirl them from side to side and flick them up, before continuing the pattern. Then I put a towel in their hands – and it became a washing routine: the abstract had gone. They started to 'do' washing. In Alexander Technique we experiment between the abstract movement and the application. When we focus on application we often bring emotional history and habit with us. In the abstract we can bring more attention to the self, how we are moving, and to our environment, the world around us.

Attention to the Environment

Despite our best endeavours, we are often only aware of the narrowed visual field right in front of us, as though we had blinkers on. I once had a client who had a pain in her foot (from tango dancing). She was a family court judge with a lot of responsibilities, and as she stood there I could see the frown and perceive her narrow focus. As we worked, I asked her to widen her gaze so she could see the honeysuckle plant to her left. She was amazed that she hadn't noticed it before. Three days into her course of lessons, the pain in her foot had gone! As we change our attention, our physical-use patterns also change.

Widening Your Gaze

We've widened your experience of the body from one part to the whole, now let's apply that to the visual field. Look at something that is directly in front of you, then move your eyes and turn your head and look at all the other things to the left and right of you, above you, on the floor and behind you. Take it all in. Now look front again and, without turning or deliberately moving your eyes or head, just allow your gaze to widen. Like opening the barn doors on a spotlight. Often when we concentrate we tighten the eyes forward and towards each other and frown. So think instead of your eyes coming back and away from each other. Can you see more now? Maybe some tension has released a little? It's useful to remember that if your eyes are open, you cannot help but see. Light comes into the front of the eye and the visual signals travel to the back of the brain where they are processed. Our eyes *are* at the back of our head! Remember our eyes move gently and subtly all the time giving us that twinkle. In any given moment we only have a visual field the size of a postage stamp. The rest of our visual perception is made up from recent past memory. You may even have a curious sense of seeing behind you. Practise deliberately narrowing your visual field and then allowing it to widen. Astonishing, isn't it? Just through paying attention differently. Perhaps you will also find that when the eyes are relaxed, you can focus more easily and see more clearly.

I have used our visual acuity to play with as we are mostly visually dominant creatures. But as you pay attention to the outside world in this gentle, more expansive way, you will also find that you become more sensitive to sounds, scents and the touch of the world.

Spatial Awareness

You can also widen your attention to include a greater spatial awareness, so important for actors, and an incredibly powerful tool to take us up and out of our habits. Spatial awareness is not something we usually think of directly. We take it for granted. But if we had no sense of the relationship in space between ourselves and other objects, the three-dimensionality of the world, we would be bumping into things.

Read through the following, carrying out the instructions as you read. If you are in a pair or group you could take it in turns to read aloud, one sentence at a time.

Taking Your Space

As you sit there, become aware of the distance between the top of your head and the ceiling. If you are outside, it will be the top of your head and the stars – eternity itself. At the same time (no cherry-picking!) become aware of the space between your back and the wall behind, between your right side and the wall to the right, your left side and the wall to the left, and the distance between you and that which is in front. It's cumulative, so eventually you will be aware of all the space around you. Add to that a sense of support from the ground through your sitting bones and your feet. The planet herself is supporting you. When we think spatially our brain starts to calm, to come down from the adrenalin-fuelled high. When we think spatially we begin to expand into the space that is there for us. Beware of 'spacing out', however: if you think only of space, you're likely to walk around like someone auditioning for *Shaun of the Dead*. It's another narrowed attention. Instead have lively eyes, receiving the details of the world around as well as the space you are living in.

As I have refined my spatial awareness over the years, I can more easily find that balanced state we want as our centre; the neutral mask, that place of potential for action that is present, calm, out of habit, aware, not concentrated, not daydreaming, not panicking about the future, just being here, now. Responsive, easy, light, effortless, where everything functions well. I offer it to you, too.

One student I was working with found it very difficult to gain any sense of the space behind her. I leaned against her back for a minute or two to stimulate her kinaesthetic sense, and then gently inched away. I stopped when she couldn't feel me any more. We practised this every lesson to help her get used to sensing the space behind her. Try it for yourself.

Finding the Space Behind

Lean against a wall with your feet about three inches away from its base. Don't try to be straight, just sense the wall supporting you in your upper back and bottom. Don't try to push your whole back against the wall or lean your head into it, just a gentle leaning, with your knees slightly bent. Then, slowly, slowly, lean away from the wall, head and chest leading – don't push your hips forward to lead – and gently, slowly walk away. How far can you get before the sense of the wall has disappeared? If you are in a pair or a group, lean against each other, back to back, for a minute or two (it's best if you are the same height, so that your backs are more in contact with each other), then have one of you move away. Stop when you no longer have the sense of the other person behind you. Is it more present for you now, the space behind? Another way of thinking about it is to imagine you are trapped in polite conversation with someone at a party and the person you fancy is behind you. There's a lot of 'back awareness' going on then!

I first came across spatial awareness whilst in rehearsal for Ibsen's play *The Lady from the Sea*, in which I was playing Ellida, the main character. Directed to remember that I was outside, looking out over fjords, I felt myself physically rise and expand into this space as my actor's imagination worked. Another time, in musical theatre, I was teaching a very tall lad in a very small room with a low ceiling. He had a habit of dropping his neck, and I was doing my best to help him find his full height. It happened to be a nice day, so we went outside into the yard and suddenly – vroom! Up he came, tall as you like. He'd been reacting to the walls and ceiling of the building hemming him in. Next time we had to work in that tiny space, I asked him to think beyond the walls, beyond the ceiling, to think of the space right up to the stars, and of the space behind, extending all the way to Chiswick Park and beyond. He didn't let the room shrink him any more.

I was taught this spatial awareness in my Alexander training as I learned to put hands on people to direct them out of their habits. 'Where is your attention, Pen? Have you got the space behind you? How about the space above?' Spatial awareness went hand in hand with a widened attention. Curiously, during my training I discovered on my own bookshelf a battered copy of *A Life of One's Own* by Marion Milner. (I had never noticed it before: how had it arrived on my bookshelf? I have no idea!) Written in 1934 and contemporary with Alexander, it's Marion's own story of discovering what would bring her to a state of happiness. And you know what it was? Widening her attention!

> 'When I considered my observations in the light of this idea of wide and narrow attention, it occurred to me that there must be two quite different ways of perceiving. Only a tiny act of will was necessary in order to pass from one to the other, yet this act seemed sufficient to change the face of the world, to make boredom and weariness blossom into immeasurable contentment.' Marion Milner[4]

And it was with delight that I read some years later of research done by Les Fehmi in the 1970s.[5] He was experimenting with volunteers to find the alpha state – a brainwave, the rate of electrical activity in the brain that is indicative of a relaxed alertness such as you might find in meditation. He was using electroencephalography (EEG), placing electrodes on the scalp to monitor brain activity. He prompted the students to think of various relaxing things – waterfalls, rose petals, peaceful landscapes, soothing sounds, and so on. These had some mild effects, but as soon as he asked them to think of the space between things, the alpha waves appeared instantly. As we think of non-doing, or of 'no-thing' such as space, the brain can go on holiday. It can release itself from thinking of Some-Thing as it thinks of No-Thing. The Taoists call this effortless action, this state of non-doing, 'Wu wei'. Alexander is not a spiritual discipline, but of all those I have come across, I consider it nearest to Taoism, with a little bit of Buddhist philosophy thrown in for good measure.

Attention to Our Activity

Different activities require different sorts of attention. When we are hunting or being hunted our adrenalin takes over; our heart beats faster, the electrical circuits in our brain rev up, our vision narrows as we target our prey or our escape. There is urgency, a driving force, to catch that thing ahead of us, to survive, no time to think of anything else: a single-minded purpose. This high-adrenalin state is literally 'exciting' our nervous system, and is thrilling. Childhood games of chase replicate this natural high and, for the most part, in the playground they are joyous, thrilling affairs accompanied by shrieks and squeals. We play at experiencing danger, and when the game is over we return to our calm learning state. The heart rate goes down, our vision widens, we laugh, we breathe more slowly, our brainwaves slow, we go back to our default mode of easy, relaxed alertness. But as we get older we begin to get stuck in the high-energy state. We become addicted to it, society encourages it, and the hunter/hunted mode becomes our default. Instead of being thrilled and excited we become stressed, anxious and fearful. We are slightly ahead of ourselves all the time, not very present. We have forgotten how to switch off, or if we do switch off, we close down from our surroundings and go into our own head.

After a lioness has finished hunting and eaten her fill of zebra, she sits quietly, relaxed but with a wide gaze, alert to any threat.

'What is this life if, full of care,
We have no time to stand and stare?'

In his poem 'Leisure', W. H. Davies is referring to staring as observing, taking in the beauty of the world around:

'No time to see, when woods we pass
Where squirrels hide their nuts in grass:

No time to see, in broad daylight,
Streams full of stars, like skies at night'[6]

We need this widening of our attention to be our centre, our default state.

Port and Starboard

Find a large room or a space outside where you can run. Exercise is always permitted!

Run as fast as you can to the opposing wall or tree. Time yourself and see if it's possible to run faster. Go again! This is hunter mode. If there are two of you, compete with each other. If there are more than two of you, make it an elimination game: name one side of the room Port and the opposing wall Starboard, whilst 'Hit the decks!' means hurling yourself flat on the floor. Have one of you call out 'Port', 'Starboard' or 'Hit the decks', and whoever gets there last is eliminated. Plenty of adrenalin going on there. And where was the attention?

Now let's change the rules. Instead of the last person being eliminated, now it's the first person to arrive. If you're on your own, move as slowly as you can from standing to lying flat out on the floor. If you are in a pair, compete to see which of you can get to the floor last. And the same for the group – caller calls out 'Hit the decks' and whoever gets there first will be out. An additional rule is that you all have to travel in the same direction and keep moving. (One round of this will be enough or it will take all day for the group to be eliminated one by one!) Where was the attention?

Change the rules again. This time both the first and the last to get there will be eliminated. For the group or the pair, call the opposing wall. If you are working on your own, walk or run without rushing, do not go slowly, do not go speedily. Where was your attention?

Was the attention different during those games? I suspect you will find that in the first elimination game, your attention narrowed to the opposing wall or tree, to running as fast as you could, targeted. When the rule changed to not being first to arrive and everything slowed down, you had more time to focus your attention on yourself and how you were doing it, perhaps also time to notice other people. And in the third game, your attention was more widespread, responding to the outside world, the other people, in a unified field of attention.

Being Present. Being Open

Alexander called the goal-orientated thinking 'end-gaining'. Intentions and desires are important, otherwise we might go round in circles, but it's good to balance our attention so that we can be aware of how we carry out those intentions. This is being attentive to our process; being present. When we allow the future and the world to come to us, we are receiving it, responding to it. Our initiative is created through our receiving. Once we find that non-striving mind, it's incredibly powerful.

One morning I was driving to college and got stuck in the usual traffic jam on Marylebone Road. My mind was churning obsessively over a problem I had with my computer. Then something brought me out of this cloud of thought for a moment and I thought 'Pen, what is it you are teaching this week? Being present? Wanting to be where you are? Practise what you are teaching!' So I began to notice what was around me: the blue sky above the buildings to my right, the shadows of trees making a pattern on the back of the large white van in front, the sound of my radio, other people in the cars next to me who I smiled at. I found myself thinking that although I wouldn't have chosen to be in a traffic jam, since that was the only way to get to college that morning – and I really wanted to be in college – I really wanted to be where I was. As I sat there enjoying the moment, it came into my mind that I had to see a student called Mark about an assignment, but I wasn't due to teach him and didn't know how to find him. Like a cloud, it just passed through my mind. I came to the end of the traffic jam and got to college in good time.

That morning I got my class to go and find five things in the building they'd never seen before – to see the place with fresh eyes, the beginner's mind. After ten minutes, four of them returned carrying Mark, saying 'Here is a zombie we've never seen before,' and laid him at my feet. I gave him the message about his assignment and he left the room. I was amazed! All that day, as I was teaching and practising present attention, doors would open for me, the sun that was troubling me would go behind a cloud, the traffic lights turned green in my favour. I can't remember what happened about the computer. I probably took it to my repair shop and it got fixed. It became less important! Sometimes things happen in our favour without our trying or making an effort, like we've allowed them into our life. We've allowed space for these things to happen.

That doesn't mean we should never take action towards a goal, but just not to narrow our attention to it. Apparently, if you want to trap a monkey, put a banana in a cage with a narrow opening. The monkey will slip his hand into the cage and grasp the banana in his fist. Then he can't take his hand out. He is trapped. He has to let go of the banana to free himself, but he won't give up that banana even though there are other bananas hanging from a tree nearby. So let's not get caught in the monkey trap. Let's widen our attention and be open to other possibilities, perhaps better ones. Often our intentions and desires are born from our habitual state. When we are in our open present state, we may not have the same desire.

Time for us to let go of narrowed, fixed attention and return to a SEA of consciousness, a unified field of attention, with time to stand and stare.

Changing Perceptions Again

The Travelator

First, raise your hand and look at the palm. Keep looking at the palm of your hand as you turn on the spot for a while. What you will see is the world spinning around whilst you appear to be still. Now keep turning but take your eyes to the world beyond your hand. Now you will perceive yourself turning. The action was the same in both cases, but you changed your perception.

Walk towards the opposite wall, or a tree or some feature in front of you. As you walk, begin to perceive the wall or the tree coming towards you. It is coming towards you, of course, because you are walking. But it is as though you are walking on the spot and the landscape is moving around you. Perhaps you will notice the wall going past you, the ground going past beneath you. This is a good one to practise in a corridor, where two walls are going past and the door in the distance is coming towards you. You may have to do this several times before you gain that different perception. If this works for you, take on another perception and imagine the future coming towards you: arriving at the door in the distance is your future, unless something else occurs unexpectedly. So now you are moving in a space–time continuum. The past is wherever you started walking from, the future where you are walking to, and the only present moment is the moment of your walking. The end of this sentence will arrive... Often people find that walking becomes easy, effortless and floaty. And seen from the outside, the person carrying out this experiment is no longer hunched, slouched or tensed up and hurrying, but walking tall with ease, grace and presence. Result! It is easy to practise this any time you are walking somewhere.

If this unified field of attention that we have been exploring here feels familiar to you, it may be that, as actors, you will already have experienced it whilst performing. As you play your role, your character is aware of other characters and the play's environment; you, as the actor, are aware of other actors, the stage and the technical crew, but also of where your props are, where the camera is and where the audience is watching you from. You may also remember that during the notes session the director asked you to hit that spot whilst delivering that line, give it a lingering pause and to be more bewildered in your response, etc. All of this is going on at the same time. It's a widened attention. So maybe I could just ask you to switch on your actor's attention?

Meantime, here are some assignments to be going on with. Enjoy the present!

Assignments

- Semi-supine: on my website I have an audio recording of me guiding your thoughts as you lie down, using spatial awareness. Please feel free to download this recording and experiment with it at least once this week if you can: www.alexanderpen.co.uk/about-the-alexander-technique/the-balanced-resting-state/

If you have trouble downloading the recording you can always make your own. In Appendix A, I have written out the text for this and you can use it in a group session, live or online, one person reading it out, whilst the others lie down in semi-supine.

- Keep a log of what your clouds of thought are and where your mind-wanders take you.

- Cataloguing: talk through what you see, hear, sense and are doing.

- Colours: each day allow a different colour into your life. If today you allowed yourself to notice blue, tomorrow could be yellow, etc.

- Practise being aware of part of yourself and to gradually widen your attention into the whole self, and the environment around.

- Practise a widened visual attention, releasing the eyes.

- The Travelator: walk as though things are coming towards you, as though the future is coming towards you.

- Practise spatial awareness.

- Make some notes on your findings.

'We must cultivate, in brief, the deliberate habit of taking up every occupation with the whole mind, with a living desire to carry each action through to a successful accomplishment, a desire which necessitates bringing into play every faculty of the attention. By use, this power develops and it soon becomes as simple to alter a morbid taste which may have been a lifelong tendency as to alter the smallest of recently acquired bad habits.' F. M. Alexander[7]

'The thing is not to try to localise the mind anywhere, but let it fill up the whole body. When this happens, you use the hands when they are needed, you use the legs, or the eyes when they are needed and no time or no extra energy will be wasted.' D. T. Suzuki[8]

Lesson Three: Alexander's Technique

Alexander's story and principles

Equipment

- Five litres of water or five kilograms of potatoes
- Space in which to speak and walk
- A long mirror
- A4 paper
- Coloured pens
- A device with internet access

How was the week of experiments in thinking? Please reflect or share in your pair or study group. These thinking experiments are for you to continue to work with throughout the course.

What was your favourite kids' game? The Farmer's in His Den? Grandmother's Footsteps? In a playful way they help improve our coordination and attention. Remember Simon Says? The leader calls out actions preceded by the words 'Simon says'. If a child obeys a command when these words are omitted, they are eliminated. It demonstrates how our brains create a prediction very quickly. The mind gets caught in a routine and stops paying full attention. (Feel free to play this game if you are in a group to remind yourselves!) In the late 1920s there were experiments made on workers' productivity in the Western Electric factory in Hawthorne, Chicago. They changed the lighting level in the workspace and productivity went up. They turned it down again, and productivity still went up. It was the change and the attention, rather than the lighting itself, that affected the workforce.[1]

How was semi-supine, using spatial awareness as recorded on the audio link on my website, or just guided by your own thoughts? Did you find that, in thinking spatially, you were more present, and as a consequence your physical tensions eased, so that your neck and shoulders freed up, your back felt longer and wider, and your limbs felt connected whilst freer and less held?

Brain Power

When we think about something it affects our brain and our muscles: there is a kinaesthetic connection. An experiment was carried out with three groups over five days to measure brain changes in learning a five-finger exercise on the piano.[2] The control group was taught the exercise and instructed not to practise. Group One was taught the exercise and instructed to practise every day for two hours. Group Two was taught the exercise and instructed to practise by sitting at the piano for two hours every day but only imagining the movements and the sounds. At the end of five days, the group who had physically practised were much more competent. But those who had imagined it had only to do two hours' physical practice on day five to level the score with Group One. The motor cortex in the brain had already changed physically to accommodate this new skill and it took only two hours for the muscles to catch up. Needless to say, the control group were not skilled at all. So as you lie in present awareness, spatially aware, asking your neck to be free to let the head release from the spine, and to allow the back to lengthen and widen, and the limbs to be long and connected, you are preparing the way for it to be so.

However, even if your mind wandered and you thought of tense-making things, your spine would still be lengthening infinitesimally and having a rest. Between the vertebrae of your spine are discs, which are rings of cartilage with a nucleus of fluid in the middle. With the weight of the head no longer bearing down, the nuclei plump up – rather like gym balls do when you've been sitting on them and then roll off them to stand. So it's nice to know that, even if all we can manage is to lie there and observe our brain in high-octane charging about, and even if we cannot feel it or are not encouraging it, something is nonetheless changing in us.

So we've sorted out the nature of habits and different ways of thinking, and are using semi-supine to help long-term in rebooting the system. Now we are prepped to have an overview of Alexander's technique to stop himself losing his voice, to understand the development of something he called the Primary Control, and to practise working with this.

Playing with Alexander's Habit

Imitating Alexander's Use

Use a line or two of text that you know well. Stand up and present this. If you are working in a group, do it all together at the same time. Now stand deliberately with the legs braced, the back arched and the chest raised, then tip the face up and pull the chin in, taking the head back and down. You will find the neck is tightened and the larynx depressed – very Edwardian. Now suck in some breath before you start and speak the text again. How was that? You may feel it was not so comfortable, the voice slightly caught, or maybe you will feel it to be rather like the way you do it already? Now let all that go and speak the text again. Did you notice there was more breath, more resonance, that you were less held, with more movement and ease throughout your body?

When we stop doing something, it's rather like thinking of space: we're not 'doing' anything, our brain stops end-gaining and we use ourselves more easily. Rather like coming out of character. We stop being Ophelia or Hamlet, and find ourselves back with ourselves very easily. We don't have to 'do' that. I just gave you the instructions that introduced you crudely to Alexander's habit of speaking as he describes it in Chapter One of his book *The Use of the Self*.[3] If you enjoy reading, find a copy and read his story from the horse's mouth, as it were. It shows you the tortuous route of his investigations into the vocal habit that was causing him to lose his voice, and how he eventually managed to inhibit the neural pathways and liberate himself. Of course, it's easier to liberate ourselves from someone else's use patterns than our own. Let's play with his technique so we can apply it to our own use patterns. This is an overview, my best attempt at summarising his method. We will be taking it apart and playing with different aspects of it throughout this course, so by the end of these eleven weeks you will have a better understanding and be able to apply the work more easily to yourself.

We've already established how important thinking is. How thinking about doing a five-finger exercise is almost as good as carrying it out. Alexander discovered that if he did nothing but think his neck free to let his head rise forward and up, in such a way that his back could lengthen and widen and his knees release – so they were not braced back and towards each other but released forward and away from each other – it brought him out of his holding pattern. He stopped pulling his head back and down, depressing his larynx and audibly sucking in the air, and he stopped arching or narrowing his back and bracing his legs, which was shortening his stature. He called these messages from the brain to the various parts of the body 'orders' or 'directions'. Just like actors being directed onstage, he was directing the play of himself. And we know that a good director does not get up onstage and show the actors how to do it, but simply guides them, allowing the actors to respond. So when Alexander had an impulse to speak, he refused and instead gave himself direction.

Directing Yourself

Alexander's Directions

Okay, your turn – have a go. Have the text in your mind, but instead of speaking, direct yourself: think these messages from the brain to the parts involved. Rather like baking a cake: for it to rise well, we have to follow the order of the recipe. So here they are in order:

'Allow the neck to be free,
so that the head can go forward and up

in such a way that the back lengthens and widens
and the knees go forward and away.'

When Alexander felt this was happening, he would then speak the text. So when you believe you are able to maintain these directions, speak your text. Did you manage to maintain ease of balance of your head, the length and width of your back? Are your legs braced or free? How do you know? Are you trusting those dodgy feelings?

Whilst, with practice, Alexander could maintain the directions as he stood preparing to speak, he eventually realised that, despite his best endeavours and feeling everything was okay, at the critical moment he went to speak the old neural pathways kicked in: he pulled his head back and down, depressed his larynx, sucked in his breath and shortened his stature as before. So he had to trick his brain to continue with the alternative way he had created. He gave himself an alternative action. He gave himself a ploy whereby he didn't have to speak, but instead could take another action – such as raising his arm. The other action has to be a real one: imagining eating a strawberry ice cream, for example, won't do.

Alexander's Inhibition

1. Decide on a line or two of text and speak it.

2. Having spoken it once to remind yourself, now think of the directions: I'm allowing the neck to be free, to let the head go forward and up, to let the back lengthen and widen, and the knees to go forward and away,' and continue to think of them as you speak the line of text.

3. Think the directions again, and just as you are about to speak the line of text, don't! Change your mind. Just stand there thinking the directions.

4. Continue to think the directions, and just as you are about

to speak the line of text, don't! Change your mind again and instead take a step backwards.

5. Continue to think the directions, and just as you are about to speak the line of text, don't! Make a choice – to stand still, to walk backwards or to speak. Play with these choices a few times.

Getting the idea? All very well, but the audience wouldn't be too pleased if, when they were expecting 'The raven himself is hoarse...' Lady Macbeth chose to walk off the stage or just stood there not doing anything. So here is the next stage:

6. Continue to think the directions, and just as you are about to speak the line of text, don't! Ask yourself if you are free to walk backwards – and if you are free to walk backwards, then you are free to speak the line of text.

Repeat this a few times, until you become familiar with it. Here are the abbreviated instructions:

Directions, about to speak, STOP, free to walk backwards? Yes! Then speak...

Record the exercise and watch it back.

If you are in a live study group, have one half do the exercise whilst the other watches, then swap. Perhaps have someone from the watching half lead the exercise. This works for a pair too. Have the appointed leader give the instructions, and let the hands clap as a stimulus to speak. I love watching a group do this – it looks like a strange fringe-theatre event at the Edinburgh Festival Fringe!

Did that have an effect on the voice, on the breath, on the stature, on how you said the line? Sometimes when people begin a new use they forget the line – it was learned under different kinaesthetic circumstances (the old habit) so the memory for a moment is lost.

By inhibiting your reaction to the stimulus to speak and giving yourself a free choice – in the present moment and not end-gaining – the old neural pathway is aborted and, after some practice and repetition, a new association is built up so that the new neural pathway can continue to be applied whilst speaking.

> 'Two roads diverged in a wood and I –
> I took the one less travelled by,
> And that has made all the difference.'
>
> Robert Frost, 'The Road Not Taken'[4]

If this is as clear as mud we will, as I wrote earlier, be spending the next few weeks unpicking it, carrying out experiments to help you understand and find your own way out of old use patterns that no longer serve you as a performer. Inhibition and direction are keys to the work.

> 'As long as he inhibits the sending of the old messages the old lines of communication are not used, and as he becomes more and more versed in the procedures of the technique the tendency to make use of them decreases, as does his dependence upon his feeling of rightness associated with them.' F. M. Alexander[5]

Heads Up

For Alexander, the dynamic relationship between the head, neck and back was very important. He called it the Primary Control. He developed the idea that, no matter what the habitual use pattern, if the neck was freed to allow the head to find its intrinsic balance, the habitual pattern would be eliminated throughout the system. There is no scientific evidence for this as yet, although there are ongoing investigations into it. But I would say we can agree that we are a whole system and that one part always affects another. So let us explore the head–neck–back relationship and see if it helps you as actors to speak well and clearly, as you make full use of the breathing mechanisms, free the jaw and make the most of the resonant space of the oral cavity and pharynx. Alexander used to pull his head back and down, hence his particular direction for the head to go forward and up. Pulling the head into the spine will distort it. Arching the back to stick the chest up will compromise the ribs and the diaphragm. Bracing the legs will pull on the diaphragm.

Let me ask you first, how much does your head weigh? Say you were playing the executioner who chops off the head of Anne Boleyn in a film and raising it by the hair to prove it was severed, what weight would you need to convey? Find five litres of water, or five kilograms of potatoes, put them in a bag, pick it up for a moment or pass it around. That's how heavy the head is. We never feel the weight of our own head. We may get a slight sense of it if, as we nod off, our head drops forward and jerks back up to wake us. It's extraordinary to think it could be that heavy. And it's right at the top of us. If the head is not resting well on top of the spine, our neck muscles will be working harder to hold it up. No wonder our neck and shoulders ache sometimes.

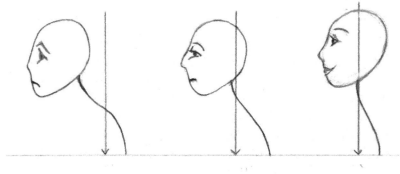

Equivalent to 19kg   Equivalent to 14.5kg   Equivalent to 5kg

Where Does Your Head Meet Your Neck?

Where does your neck end and head begin? Just point to where you think that is...

I bet you have put your finger somewhere at the back of your neck. It's harder to think of it from the front. But know that, if you could see through your face, the top vertebra of your spine would be like a moustache on your upper lip. If you place your fingertips in the groove behind your jaw, up by the ear on both sides, that is the nearest you can get to touching the front of the top of your spine. And the skull rests just behind that groove. You could try touching the front of your spine by opening your mouth and sticking your finger to the back of your throat, but it has unfortunate gagging consequences. So find a mirror, open your mouth and look at the murky depths behind the uvula. That is skin covering the front of the spine. If you stick one finger in the groove as before and one finger as far into the mouth as it will go before gagging, you will get a really good idea of where your spine meets your skull. Put both fingers in the groove each side again and gently nod your head up and down, turn it slightly from one side to the other and make circles in the air with your nose. Make these movements very, very small so the main neck muscles are not activated. You will be sensing the atlanto-occipital (AO) joint working, and also the atlanto-axial (AA) joint. That's where your head moves on the spine, and where the first vertebra, the atlas, rotates on the second, the axis. These joints are unlike any of the other vertebrae of your spine. They are freely movable joints with synovial fluid between them, just like the joints of your limbs. (The rest of the vertebrae in the spine have cartilaginous joints; discs between them which, whilst allowing distortion, are much less movable.)

You will get some great 3D images and videos of this on the internet. You could get out your phone now and have a look, or search for one as part of your assignment for this week. In the meantime, here's a static illustration:

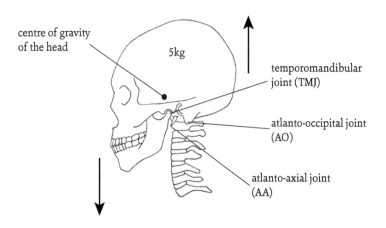

The cervical spine in the neck has 80-degree rotation to both sides, the thoracic spine has 30–40-degree rotation and the lumbar spine about 5–7 degrees. The head can be freely movable on your spine. If you look at the side of the head you will notice that there is still more head in front of the spine than behind. The balance point is an unequal fulcrum so, obeying the laws of gravity, the face or front of the head is gently dropping downwards all the time, which raises the back of the head up. It doesn't drop all the way, bending the neck, because small, sensitive muscles around the AO and AA joints change length all the time to keep it balanced, as well as the large muscles of the neck acting like guy ropes on a tent – all dynamically changing to allow movement of the head. It has potential energy because it is about to fall. When the neck tightens and pulls the head into the spine, the potential energy has gone.

I like to think of an image from an early physics class: a rock has potential energy when it is about to fall from a cliff, teetering on the edge. If it is stuck there and solidly attached to the cliff it is inert and it would take some effort to push it off. We want effortlessness! When the head is tipped back for any length of time it feels wrong and it is a strain on the muscles – you are having to use effort as they tense and shorten themselves. Feel this on yourself. Let your nose drop a little and sense how the back of your head rises a little. This is different from dropping your neck down; it's just a small dropping motion of the head, not the neck. You may feel this even more if you release your jaw a little. The jaw is so often held tightly up against the skull, pushing it up and back. It's really useful to explore these top two joints with another person: feeling it on someone else will give you a really good idea of how it works in you. If you are working alone, read the instructions below and make it part of your assignment this week to find someone to play with, if possible.

Balancing the Head

In pairs, have one sit in the chair and the other stand at the side. The one standing cups their hands on the other's forehead and the back of the head. The one sitting looks down at their lap and then looks up and back at the ceiling. The one sitting has control of their own head all through this exercise. The one standing is just following and sensing the movement with their hands. Swap round and discuss. Doesn't it feel like the head is about to come off its rockers as the other person looks up and back? Not a balance you want to stay in for long!

Now have one sit down on a chair and the other stand behind. The one standing places the tips of their index fingers in the groove behind their partner's jaw, and asks them to nod gently up and down, from side to side, and to do little circles with their nose. Then they place the tips of the little fingers in the groove and place the other fingers on the head above the ear. They ask the one sitting to look at something all the way to the right and then all the way to the left, so they can feel the head turning. The one sitting will also be reminded of where the head is turning from because the little fingers are nearly touching those joints. Now let the head turn again but this time the one standing leads the movement. They will find the head turns very easily if their partner is allowing them to move it gently. Swap it round. And discuss.

Compare this way of turning the head from the top joints with turning it lower down. Just for a moment, drop your neck as though you were looking at your phone – 'tech neck', as it is sometimes called. Keep the neck there, dropping forward, but tilt your head up so you can see what is in front of you. Now turn your head from side to side. How do you rate that in terms of ease? Now look up at the ceiling. Think of lengthening up through the front of you as you tilt your head back a little way. Open your jaw and, using the AO joint as a pivot, allow your head to come up and over to meet the jaw. You may feel your head rising up and rebalancing itself nicely, and the spine lengthening as it is freed from the weight of the head. Now turn your head from side to side from there. Easier? This is a very good movement to play with if you are in doubt as to where the head should be in order to be in balance. Just mapping where the head meets the spine can make an enormous difference to how you use yourself.

Mapping the Neck and Jaw

Having an accurate body map changes the way you perceive yourself and makes your direction much more accurate and effective. For example, when I suggest that you free your neck, what area are you thinking of? You probably have a good idea of where the back and sides of your neck are, but the front is an interesting region. We know now that it extends up to that 'groove', but how far does it go down? In a way it segues into the shoulders. I like to think of it ending at the top of the ribs just above the collarbone and the shoulder blades. But if we think of the trapezius muscle, the top of which can get very stiff either side of the neck and shoulders, the bottom of it goes all the way down to the middle of the back at the T12 vertebra

– a good leverage point to stop the head falling forward with gravity. So if you think of the trapezius as part of the neck, it makes a big difference when you ask your neck to be free. You are paying attention to, and directing, a bigger area.

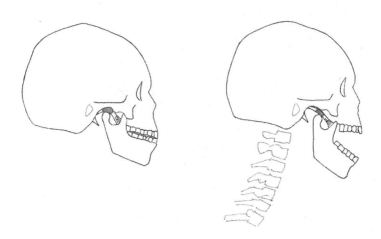

The front of the neck includes the jaw. The jaw is also part of the face, jointed to the skull. Place the flat of your hand at the joint of your jaw, the temporomandibular joint (TMJ), just in front of your ear, and open and close your jaw a few times. You will feel that the joint slides forward first and then hinges open. It also has the ability to move from side to side for chewing. For our purposes it is enough to know that it slides forward and down to open, up and back to close. Knowing that can, again, make the movement easier, more conscious. It is easier to release the jaw if you know the action of the joint. If you are only trying to hinge it, it will add tension rather than releasing it. Try hinging deliberately – feel how it pulls the jaw into the throat?

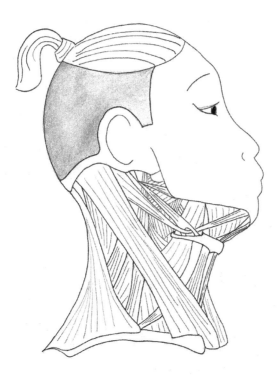

The muscles around there are flexible but also very strong. We open the jaw to release the voice, and we close it to chew savagely on our food. As we release the jaw we release the neck, so we could think of the jaw as part of the neck rather than the head. So as you free your neck – the huge area including trapezius down to T12 and the jaw – the head is released forward and up out of the spine into that balance of potential energy. There are over sixty muscles in the neck. It would be impossible to direct each individual muscle – they do not move individually but are moving in sequence, as a team. Do you know the poem about the happy centipede who was rendered incapable of movement by a toad who asked her which leg moved after which?[6] Alexander never suggested we get into that sort of detail – a simple direction to an area sufficed. But knowing something of where and how that area moves can help enormously. Isn't it great to know we've got so many muscles in the neck helping us move and support the head, the larynx, the tongue and the jaw, so we can speak and chew and turn and duck and gaze up at the stars? And we don't have to pull on them. They are happily able all by themselves to release and free up to allow movement. Some muscles will be getting shorter, others will be lengthening, contracting and releasing in sequence to ensure easy movement. I was always taught at school that muscles contract. The opposing muscles would be releasing but I understood it to be a passive response to the contraction. However, I have learned through my Alexander practice that if, instead, we pay attention to the release and lengthening of the muscles, then the contraction will happen effortlessly with just the right amount of tension.

The jaw is at the front of the neck, and is also the bottom of the face. The face is not the head. When learning to swim as a little girl, I was asked to hold my breath and dip my head under the water. I leant over and put my face in the water. My teacher guffawed and, putting his hand on the top of my head, dunked me. It was a revelation. That was my whole head submerged in water. Ah–ha! (It also helped me learn to swim.) Often, if I suggest to a new student that they think of the head going up, they will take their face up. Just for a moment, tip your face up. What happens? As the face goes up, the head goes back and down – the opposite of what is required. So sometimes I will direct someone to let the face drop in order to let the back of the head rise. Just for a moment, get to know the dimensions of your head. Place the palms of your hands on your forehead and the back of your head. Then place them on the sides of your head, just above your ears, and now place one hand on the top of your head and one on the back of your head. Got it? Now you are clear on this, you can have a free neck and jaw with a head that is well balanced, obeying the laws of gravity, and allowing the back to lengthen and widen.

The Back and Spine

Drawing Your Back

How do you perceive your back? What's in it? Where does it begin and end? Think about this for a moment. Draw a picture of your back – with your left hand as in Lesson One, if you like. It's just to find a representation of your understanding of the back. Reflect on this drawing or discuss it with a partner. Do you include the pelvis in the back? The shoulders? Keep your drawing and put in your logbook.

I think we can all agree there is a spine in there somewhere. The spine continues into the neck, but is definitely part of the back – it is sometimes called the backbone, after all. It's very common to mis-map the spine. So let's pay some attention to its placement in us and our beliefs around that.

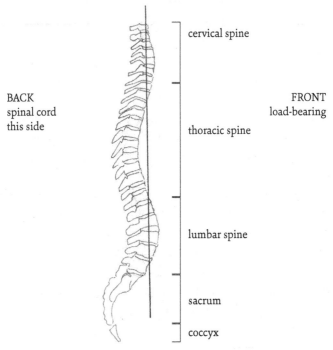

cervical spine

BACK
spinal cord
this side

FRONT
load-bearing

thoracic spine

lumbar spine

sacrum

coccyx

You will see that it is made up of bones called vertebrae which, apart from the atlas and axis at the top that we've already played with, are all stuck firmly together by cartilage – the discs – to make up one bony system. Having separate bones means it is flexible as well as being a firm supporting mechanism. As you might expect, the vertebrae at the top of your spine are smaller than the vertebrae at the bottom. Five vertebrae are welded together to form a wedge-shaped bone called the sacrum, which attaches firmly to the pelvis; and right at the end we have the coccyx – what is left of our tail, four tiny vertebrae, also fused together. For convenience we give different names to parts of the spine, but remember it is one continuous structure.

You Do Not Want a Straight Spine!

Lengthening Device

Place your hands on top of your head and let the weight of your arms take the head into the spine. Keep it there for about fifteen seconds. Now take your hands off – can you feel how the head rises? The spine is automatically lengthening: it is a lengthening device; it likes to be as long as possible. It squashes down to take the added weight and lengthens up when the weight is taken off.

The spine develops its cervical, thoracic and lumbar curves once we start walking as toddlers, adapting to the weight of the head, allowing us some 'give'. If we had no curves it would be quite painful to walk around. Our problems arise when the curves become too pronounced and we lose our bounce, becoming stuck and immovable. Our body adapts beautifully to our use. If we decide we want to keep our head ducked down and upper back curved over, it will accomplish this and make it easier for us by shortening the muscle length. When we want to change that, it will accommodate that too – but it will take some time; maybe fifteen days of continual lengthening for the muscle fibres to adapt (and it may not always feel comfortable during that shift).

The Depth of the Spine

Working in a pair, let one of you place the fingers of one hand in a line down the side of the other's neck, and the other hand at the back of the spine, where the sacrum meets the pelvis at the sacroiliac joint.

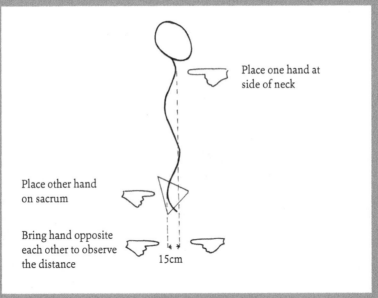

Place one hand at side of neck

Place other hand on sacrum

Bring hand opposite each other to observe the distance

15cm

Keep your hands there and ask your partner to step away. Let your top hand move gently downwards and the bottom hand rise up until the palms are opposite each other, whilst keeping the same distance from one palm to the other. You will find they are about 15cm away from each other. This is the parameter between which the spine snakes through your neck and torso. It's not that any single vertebra is that big, you understand, it's the overall width of the curves. Swap.

The Front of Your Spine is More Central Than You Realised

Looking again at the picture you will see that the weight-bearing area of the spine is at the front. At the back is the corridor the spinal cord passes along, that bundle of nerves streaming their way down to the body, transporting the messages to and from the brain.

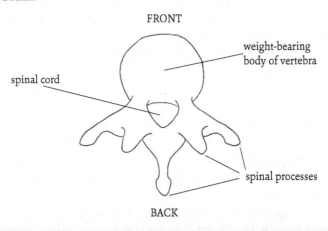

FRONT

weight-bearing
body of vertebra

spinal cord

spinal processes

BACK

Feeling the Spine

Run your fingers down the back of your spine from the top of your neck to your pelvis, as best you can. If working with a partner, feel the back of their spine. Those characteristic bumps, particularly noticeable in the thoracic region, are the spinal processes.

They are for muscle attachment and form a ring that protects the spinal cord. They are connected to each other with facet joints which allow for the flexion, extension and the twisting motion of the spine. Because we can touch our spine at the back we can get confused and assume our spine is only at the back. But the processes you are touching are not weight-bearing. It is the body of the vertebrae and the discs between them, acting like shock absorbers, that are the supporting area of the spine, and they are at the front. Let's now get in touch with that support deep within.

Thinking into the Spine

Stand up and place your hand on your own or your partner's lumbar spine and just think for moment that the front of these vertebrae are about 8cm in from where your hand is. Then stand independently, arms at your sides, gently directing yourself, thinking of the front of your own spine. Perhaps look at the picture of the spine to help your thinking. Think up from the front of the coccyx, travelling up the front of the sacrum, the front of the lumbar spine as it curves forward, the front of the thoracic spine as it curves back to make room for the heart and lungs, the front of the cervical spine as it rises up the front of your neck at the back of your mouth until it reaches the base of your skull between your ears. Then think all the way down the front of the spine, from those top two vertebrae between the ears, back of the mouth, behind the larynx, past the lungs, behind the heart, forward down the lumbar curve and back down the curve of the sacrum and coccyx. Our spine is much more central than we often believe. Does that change how you experience standing?

In my old belief system I had my spine on upside down and back to front – I thought the lumbar spine had the most rotation, the neck the least, and the support was in the bony processes at the back, with the spinal cord travelling through the front. Oops. I also had it mapped much shorter than it was.

Lengthening the Spine

Place one hand in your lumber curve, just above the pelvis, fingers pointing down. Take your other hand to the middle of the back of the neck. Keep your hands there and take a walk. This is where some imagine the spine to begin and end. Now pause and let your lower hand slide down onto the sacrum at the back of your pelvis – the end of your middle finger will be between the 'cheeks', about where the coccyx are. Place a finger of the other hand in the groove behind your ear. Keep the hands there and go for a walk. Is that a different experience?

There's More to the Back

Of course, the spine itself doesn't widen, so whilst it may be lengthening as we direct ourselves, there is more to the back than just the spine to consider. How about the shoulder blades, the ribs and the pelvis? Remember, you just had your hand on the sacrum where the spine is connected to the pelvis. Enveloping all that bony stuff is a web of muscles, ligaments and tendons that connect and organise them. Deep within are the supporting and movement muscles of the spine and the ribs.

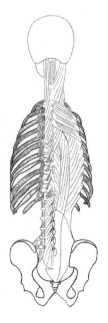

...and on the surface the muscles that organise the limbs.

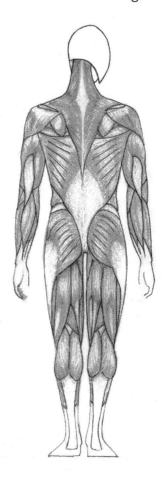

If we raise the chest, we are contracting the muscles of the lower back, narrowing it, and if we brace our legs we are contracting the muscles of our pelvis, the glutes, and again arching and narrowing the lower back. The ribs are jointed to the spine. As actors, we certainly don't want to be restricting the movement of the ribs by squeezing them together. The squeezing is carried out by muscles pushing and pulling the bones together. Bones really don't like that very much. They prefer to move freely.

If we squeeze our shoulder blades together (shoulders back, chin in, chest out!) we are narrowing the upper back. If you pat yourself on the back – and why not, I'm sure you deserve it – you are actually patting muscles functionally concerned with the arm – your arms come out of your back! As you release your shoulders, you widen the back. As you unbrace the legs, you widen the back. Come into your whole back! Pay attention to it! As we lengthen and widen the whole back, we cannot help but affect the whole system, our limbs as well.

Making sure we have an accurate map of ourselves will enable Alexander's directions to be more easily carried out. 'I'm allowing my neck to be free, so that my head goes forward and up, so that my back lengthens and widens, and my knees go forward and away.' (More on legs in the next lesson...)

Brain Maps the Body

Our brain builds up a body map of ourselves in different ways.[7] It maps the space around us as part of ourselves. (Remember the last lesson on spatial awareness?) We know this instinctively: if someone stands too close, it is uncomfortable to us – they are invading our space. As we take in the space around us, we expand into this space: we become more confident because we have enlarged our personal space. We own our space. Just what you want onstage, where your audience is being invited into your space. You are letting them come to you – just like *The Travelator*, allowing the wall or the future come to you. If we hold something in our hand, the brain maps it as if it is part of us. The walking stick is an extension of our arm, and the texture of the ground can be felt through the stick. The same is true if you are holding a pen – you can feel the texture of the paper though the pen. When we are in touch with someone else, the brain begins to read the other person as ourselves.

Another important map is the representation of the body in the motor and sensory motor cortex in the brain. The two cortexes run in parallel at the top of the brain. If you place two fingers above one ear and walk them over the top of the head to the other ear, that's the rough placement of these cortexes in your brain, the left side corresponding to the right side of the body, the right side to the left. The sensory cortex is receiving information from your body, the motor cortex is sending messages from brain to the body.

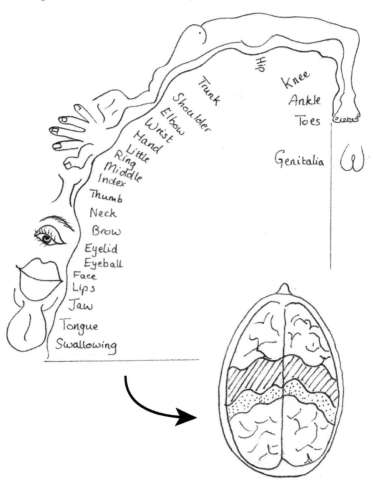

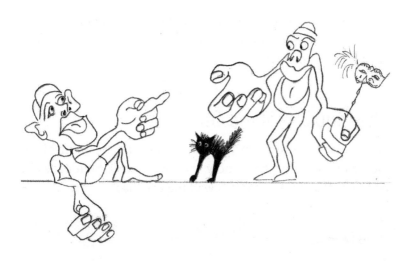

The visual representation of how the brain perceives us makes us look like a very strange gnome! The map is dependent on the number of nerve endings we have in any one part of the body. There are many more in the face and hands, so these parts are enormous compared to the back, which has fewer. Put your hand out, close your eyes and ask someone to touch it with their fingers. Guess how many fingers they used. Now ask them to do the same on your back. It's harder to know for sure, isn't it? There are less nerve endings in the back to distinguish the different fingers. In recent years neuroscience has discovered that our brains have plasticity and that repeating certain actions changes the size of that area of the cortex. Our brain changes physically to adapt to our actions.

The sort of body mapping we have been considering, however, and which is so useful in changing our habits and beliefs, was developed by Bill and Barbara Conable whilst working with musicians at the Ohio State University. Barbara now teaches body mapping as a separate discipline. I watched her work with a violinist who produced an exquisite sound simply by reconsidering where her 'violin shelf' was, how her lower arm rotated and where the joints of her fingers were. As Barbara explains it, the process of body mapping is applying the truth of anatomy to our movement, so we then move as our bodies are designed to move.[8]

The Map is Not the Territory

Let's return to experimenting with the dynamic relationship of the head, neck and back, now that you have a better idea of where it all is. Let's use it in a walking exercise.

Head Leading

As you walk, let your head lead and the rest follow. As you turn, let the head begin the rotation, and let the rest follow. If you are in a group, choose someone of a similar height, and have one of you close their eyes and the other stand behind. As when you were sitting, place the little finger in the groove and let the other fingers rest above the ear on either side of the head. Lead your partner by the head around the room. If you want them to stop, take your hands off. Otherwise you can turn them on a pin. Swap and discuss. I am suggesting your partner's eyes are closed so that there is no anticipation of where you are taking them, and they are totally reliant on you for guidance. Don't talk about it as you do this. Keep it going for a couple of minutes and then stop, discuss, and swap it round. What's your experience? Does it work? Return again to working on your own with eyes open and direct yourself to let the head lead and the rest follow.

To sum up this lesson: you had a first experience of Alexander's technique, directing himself and inhibiting his habit of speaking *before he spoke*, by giving himself options of doing something else. The directions are messages from the brain primarily to the head, neck and back, which are in a dynamic relationship. This dynamic relationship of the head, neck and back he called a Primary Control, and when they coordinate well, they liberate the voice. We investigated the notion of mapping the body and our beliefs, in particular of the head, neck and back. And experimented in walking with the head leading and the rest following. A load of new information and experiences. You will remember a lot. The assignments will help.

Assignments

- Semi-supine – vary it by using spatial thinking with or without the audio recording and using Alexander's directions. You remember that, as you lie there, these directions are already starting to happen by the very act of your lying down in semi-supine. Perhaps thinking them at the same time will enhance the process.

- Be aware of how the head sits on the spine as you go about your daily grind. Occasionally practise looking up, opening the jaw and taking the head up and over to meet the jaw to reorganise how the head sits on the spine.

- Think of the front of your spine from time to time.

- Practise walking with the head leading.

- Solo artists: when you can, find someone to let you feel the atlanto-occipital and atlanto-axial joints working as they gently nod their head up and down, side to side and do circles with their nose leading. (Pairs and groups: it will help you learn this better if you repeat the exercise with others.) Then, with your partner sitting in a chair, carry out the head-turning exercises, and then feel the movement of the head as they slowly look up and then down. Perhaps they will also let you lead them by the head in walking, as described in the last exercise. And check out the parameters of the spine with this same willing partner too, if possible.

- On the internet look up the AO and AA joints, pictures of the whole spine, and the muscles of the neck and back. Print them off and stick them up on your wall – somewhere you can see them easily. If you just leave them on your device you won't be seeing them in peripheral vision or subconsciously. I want them to be part of the wallpaper for a couple of weeks, so you don't have to study them, just become aware of them. Easy learning!

- Make notes in your logbook.

'I heard the term "use your full height". But what does that even mean: stand up straighter? I would look in the mirror and stand without applying my directions. Then keeping relaxed, think of allowing my neck to be free, so my head rises, my back lengthens and widens and my knees go forward and away. I found I looked more alert and interesting and looked more my natural height. "You've gotten taller," said one of my mates in Birmingham that holiday. "Thanks," I said.' Tom, drama student

'I tend to stick my neck out. I had noticed I stuck my neck out in performance also. When I felt particularly passionate towards something or felt I wanted to really express something in either acting or singing, it would happen. So I gave myself the task of making sure I thought about it in each different activity I did in the day for a week. This proved harder than I expected. But when I remembered, I did find that having the thought of my directions lifted me both in a physical and mental way. When feeling my back lengthening and widening there was also this sudden release of the tension from my inner thoughts, and I felt uplifted.' Rosie, drama student

'The Silken Tent'
Robert Frost[9]

She is as in a field a silken tent
At midday when the sunny summer breeze
Has dried the dew and all its ropes relent,
So that in guys it gently sways at ease,
And its supporting central cedar pole,
That is its pinnacle to heavenward
And signifies the sureness of the soul,
Seems to owe naught to any single cord,
But strictly held by none, is loosely bound
By countless silken ties of love and thought
To every thing on earth the compass round,
And only by one's going slightly taut
In the capriciousness of summer air
Is of the slightest bondage made aware.

'…for the employment of the Primary Control in my technique is inseparable from the inhibitory procedures necessary to the reconditioning of the reflexes and to integration of the "total pattern" involving the same procedures in a unified process.' F. M. Alexander[10]

Lesson Four: Walk Tall!

Experiments in walking

Equipment

- Space in which to walk and crawl
- A wall
- Filming equipment and/or mirror
- A tape measure

'When I walk seamlessly, it seems less that way.' Jamee Culbertson, Alexander teacher

You walk into auditions, walk onstage, walk onto the set, walk into frame, out of shot... Walking is quite an important part of an actor's life. The wonderful thing is, you can practise walking throughout the day, no rehearsal time necessary! Characters will have their own way of walking but let's find out what you the actor are up to, so we can change your habits of walking to find a neutral, unaccented locomotion using Alexander's method of direction and inhibition. Be prepared in this chapter to do a lot of walking in between reading the instructions!

What is your choreography for walking?

Exaggerating Your Walk

Film yourself again or look in a mirror as you perambulate by. Then have a go at exaggerating it, so you are very clear what you are doing. If you can work in pairs, have one person walk in front and the other walk behind, copying the walk. Of course, it's not just the walking motion you are observing, but the use of the whole person – are they swinging their arms, are they pulled down to one side, do they bounce, stomp, float, are they speedy or do they saunter, is their head tilted, are their shoulders hunched, do they kick with their legs? Whatever you notice, solemnly imitate this as accurately as you can for a minute and then have fun with it – exaggerate the walk so it is slightly ridiculous. Now have the walker drop out and observe the imitator, then drop back in again behind them and imitate their own exaggerated walk. Stop and discuss. And swap round, so the walkers can get their own back!

In many large tourist artistic spaces around the world, like London's Covent Garden or outside the Pompidou Centre in Paris, you'll find mime artists creating an entertainment by walking behind an unsuspecting member of the public and imitating them. It's very skilled and very funny – and, of course, they are careful to choose people who are fit to make fun of. A good assignment for you this week, maybe?

We're all walking effectively – we all get where we want to go – yet we all walk slightly differently. However, there are some general points we can play with.

Ways of Walking

Did any of you find you were bouncing, the head rising up and down as the foot pushed you up? Have a go at a walk that bounces. Any of you find that you drop into the hip, like a horse walking slowly down a hill? Have a go at walking by dropping into the hip. And then there's that lovely hip sway – a wiggle or a longer movement. Play with that one. Now walk keeping your legs straight, rolling from side to side. Now walk by kicking the foot in front as you go. How about walking with your toes turned out – how does that feel?

More Haste, Less Speed

Then there's speed. Some of us have a slower rhythm than others. I live in London, but also spend a lot of time on an island in Greece. I recognise that I am much faster paced in London – my system has got used to the gym, the 'rush' of the city and the cold climate. In Greece in the summer, the tempo is much slower and the rush disappears. '*Siga, siga*', as they say: 'Gently/slowly, gently/slowly'.

Taking the Story Out of the Walk

Walk around again and, as you do so, imagine that you are late for an appointment with a casting director: the train was delayed and your mobile is out of action so you just have to get there as quickly as possible – go! And pause. How was that? Unless you've broken into a trot, you will be using a lot of effort to get there, mostly by tightening all the muscles with urgency. Here's a secret: when we rush and strain, we actually go a little slower! Do the exercise again and at the fastest pace. Take away the rush, the story of the casting director, the stress of trying, but still walk as fast as before. Do you find that it's easier and even a little quicker?

Walking with excessive tension is like driving with the handbrake on – to be avoided, unless you enjoy the anxious, adrenalin-fuelled stomp. One of my American colleagues worked with an Olympic rowing team, and they won the gold medal. When they didn't contact him next season for further help in their training, he was surprised and rang them up. 'Gee, Tommy, we loved what you did with us, but we kind of missed the burn.'

Whether you are someone who walks with a bounce, swinging the legs, rushing or quietly idling, if it's getting you where you want to go without injury then all is well. However, as an actor it is best to find a way of moving that is graceful, free, easy, effortless and centred; less idiosyncratic, walking tall, taking your space, available for anything. So how can we achieve this?

Walk On

Let's consider in more detail some of the general habits of walking which may apply to you. We'll look at your beliefs, and try a little more body mapping to help you out.

One of the major habits people get into is stiffening the legs and trying to push the earth away. There's a belief that if we don't use all that effort to push ourselves against the force of gravity, we will collapse and fall over. But what really keeps us standing upright? The spine? The back? The legs? The balance of the head? Actually, it is the power of thought. Consciousness. If we faint, we fall over. We need to be awake, that's all. And gravity is not our foe but our friend, keeping us attached to the earth. Otherwise we would just float off into space.

We start to walk aged nine months onwards and most of us have learnt this hazardous skill by seventeen months. Before then we are desperate to get ourselves around: we roll, we squirm, we crawl and bum-shuffle, heave ourselves up with our hands, so urgent is our need to go towards the stimuli of the world around us – particularly food, and brightly coloured toys that sparkle and make weird noises. As soon as we have free will we want to walk. Hazardous, yes, but jolly convenient. Being on two legs and balancing is much easier than having to use the muscular effort of four legs. Look at a toddler, and you will see them using their knees a lot. They don't walk with straight legs. This is something we learn later, by playing football or going to ballet, perhaps, or by copying our parents.

Rock and Roll

The main joints of your legs? Hip, knee and ankle. If we stiffen these joints we cannot move freely. If you ever need to play a character that has a roll in their gait, that is how to find it – easy peasy, lemon squeezy. And if you want to eliminate the rolling gait, just free the joints of your legs – and bend your knees more! Easier said than done, of course, if it's a very ingrained habit.

When we stiffen the legs we are usually swinging the leg from the mysterious waist joint that doesn't exist. Let's check out the body map again. Without thinking too hard, just point to where you believe your hip joint to be. If you are pointing to the side or front, level with your groin, have a gold star. If you are pointing to the top of your pelvis, oh-oh! You are not alone. It is partly to do with our English language: we call the pelvis the hip, and where does the hip/pelvis end? So it must be jointed there, surely? No.

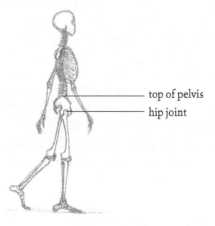

top of pelvis

hip joint

Exploring This Very Hip Joint

Where is the halfway point of your height? Not your belly button, or the top of your pelvis, but the hip joint, which sits in the groin. Your legs are about the same length as your head, neck and torso. Measure yourself to check this out. Remember this is an average and if you are very tall it is probable that your legs are longer. And make sure you measure the length of leg from the hip joint, not the top of your pelvis. Now place your thumb on the hip joint and rest your fingers on the side and top of your leg pointing downwards. Move around the room again and feel the movement of your hip joint. It is essential to become familiar with the geography of this joint. Check it out on Google or YouTube. (Be wary of the walking skeletons that come up – they are not necessarily using themselves well!) Sit and stand a couple of times, too, and you will feel how your torso bends forward from the same area. Can you feel that joint working? If you had previously believed the joint to be at the top of your pelvis, then it is likely you have been bending forward from the waist and organising your leg movement from there. Hurrah – you are now liberated from the mysterious waist joint! Just knowing where the hip joint is situated may now be altering your walking pattern. No more rock and roll. When we swing the leg from the waist we often also add a little kick to the lower leg before we place it on the floor, as though we thought the feet had to get there in advance of the head. But when the head leads, your legs will come under you to support you. When we kick our lower leg forward we are bracing and jarring the leg. (Like heel-striking when you're running – best to run more on the front of your foot to relieve the jarring.) I blame 'The Beautiful Game' for all this surreptitious kicking and swinging. Walk around like this for a while, kicking your lower leg forward. If it's not your habit you will feel the effort it takes.

A Bounce in Your Step

Now let's look at the bouncing gait.

Have a Bounce

Walk around deliberately bouncing. Instead of the head remaining level, it is being displaced, the whole of you bobbing up and down as you bounce along. It can be quite exhilarating, and we are certainly using our leg joints. But it takes a lot of energy and is again a symptom of pushing yourself away from the planet – a hidden belief that you have to 'do' walking, that without that extra push you wouldn't get anywhere. It's like a jump or hop that hasn't quite taken off, as if we have to drive ourselves forward.

Supposing, instead, we learn to tread the earth gently. Think of your knee joint for a moment. The knee is where your thigh bone and shin bone meet. We sometimes erroneously think of the knee as the kneecap. The kneecap protects the knee joint and the tendons there, it is not weight-bearing. Just move it around for a moment. You can have the kneecap removed and, although kneeling may then be uncomfortable, it won't stop you walking. A joint is always a space between the bones and is three-dimensional.

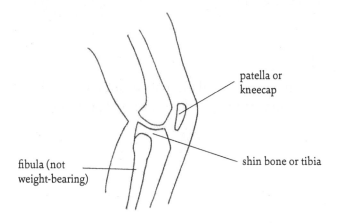

patella or
kneecap

fibula (not
weight-bearing)

shin bone or tibia

Our knee is not at the front of the leg, but at the back, too. A drama student came complaining of shin splints – pain in the shin, the lower part of the front of the leg – as he leapt up and down in a dance class. We re-mapped his image of his knee joint so he could think from the back of the knee, and his pain disappeared. Another young actor had had surgery on her knee and was afraid to bend her leg in case she injured it again. It felt tight, too. Understanding that the kneecap was not weight-bearing, and that she could receive the support of the earth through the back of her knee joint, totally relieved her of that fear and she walked easily and happily, the tightness gone. Here's a thought: as we walk, the heel peels itself off the floor, the top of the shin bone drops forward. No pushing or bouncing needed. Have a go.

Dropping Your Shin Bone

With a partner place, two fingers on the top of their shin bone and ask them to walk a couple of paces – you will feel that action of the shin bone. Then experiment for yourself. As you walk, just be aware of the top of the shin bone dropping forward, allowing the heel to peel itself off the floor. Does that shift something? Does that stop the bounce? Does it also continue to unstiffen the leg?

Walking in Turnout

I blame ballet for the perpetual turnout. Most dancers will have cultivated this from standing in first or second position.

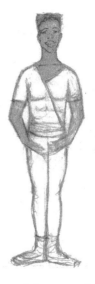

Ballet is a beautiful form of dance, originating in Renaissance Italy and spreading to the French court in the late sixteenth century. It's elegant, highly stylised and disciplined. But it is not natural to our species. When you are standing in turnout, your buttocks are contracting and your hip is being rotated so that you are able to raise your leg higher. (If you raise your leg to the side without being in turnout, it can physically only go so far before the greater trochanter meets the pelvis. Ouch!) As an actor you do not need to do this. When we walk with our feet turned out we also tend to flatten the arch of the foot. So, if walking and standing in turnout is your thing, play with not doing that.

A Parallel Universe

Stand up and turn your feet out as you walk. For the dancers amongst you, this will feel very familiar! Experiment with walking with your feet in parallel to each other. It may feel like your knees are knocking towards each other, but if you check in the mirror, they probably won't be. Be aware that this can have extraordinary consequences, like changing your whole sense of self!

A young actor once presented a piece of text he was working on for a play. He was standing in turnout and moving around in a way that was quite distracting. He said that he was speaking as the character – acting – so I asked him, just for now, drop the character and speak the text again. He was still standing in turnout, unaware that it was his habit. He agreed to stand in parallel and a look of consternation came over his face. He was transformed. He spoke the text and I heard it. No trying to get something right, just experiencing something outside of his habit, and as a result he got out of the way of himself. (Note that I am not suggesting that we all walk in parallel – it's not 'right', it's just different. I believe that if you let the leg hang, there is a natural turnout, but it's just not pronounced.)

Walking with a Wiggle

How about the swaying pelvis? The pelvis moves when we walk, coordinating with the leg movement and the swing of the arms. Although the bones of the leg attach lower down in the pelvis than perhaps you thought, the top muscles of the legs, the buttock muscles, attach to the top of the pelvis. (They are the glutes: gluteus maximus, gluteus medius and gluteus minimus – three Roman generals!) The natural sway turns into an exaggerated wiggle when we drop into the hip joint as we walk, displacing the pelvis outwards. Or if we walk with one foot in front of the other.

Less Wiggle Room

Walk with one foot in front of the other on a single line. You will feel the pelvis swaying or wiggling more. Now walk with the feet further apart in two parallel lines. Feel the difference? A generalisation would be, if you want to have a more 'girly' walk, then walk with one foot in front of the other on a single line. If you want to have a more 'boyish' walk, walk with the feet apart on two lines. The anatomy of our gender can affect our use. Now have a go at exaggerating the sway by dropping into the hip joints. As you drop into the hip joint, the corresponding leg will stiffen. Now have a go at not dropping into the joints. Different?

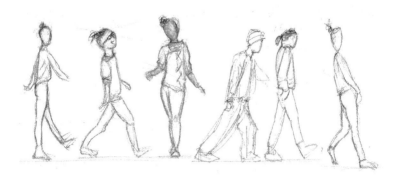

Walking in Opposition

Does the right arm move forward with the right foot? This is rare but some people have a tendency not to coordinate the limbs in opposition.

Walking without Opposition

Have a go deliberately walking with right arm and right leg together, followed by left arm, left leg. You might notice quite a fierce torque on the legs, or there may be a sideways contraction helping you move, like a lizard. The ribs drop down towards the pelvis on one side and then the other. At the same time, the pelvis is being driven up towards the ribs as the leg is braced. Again, it often occurs when the hip joint is mis-mapped in the brain and the 'waist joint' is being activated. Play instead with marching around the room in soldierly fashion. As the right leg moves forward, the left arm swings forward, and vice versa. Don't overthink or you will end up like that centipede! The spine, too, will be rotating slightly, being wound up one way and releasing the other way, creating a useful energy. It becomes more obvious when we run, the opposing limbs rotating around the spinal column, head staying centre.

Look at the drawing of the superficial muscles of the back on page 219. See how the muscle fibres of the 'glutes' lie in the same direction as the muscle fibres of the 'lats' that attach to the arm? They are separate muscles, but the fibres are coordinated to organise the arm swing and rotation. Sometimes we can think walking is just a leg action, but remember that walking developed from crawling, and the upper limb is still involved. In fact, all of us is involved in walking!

The Leading Role

As part of last week's assignments I asked you to practise walking with the head leading. But what is leading you when you are walking habitually, in your own pattern? Is there a particular part of the body that likes to get ahead of everything else? If you're not sure, ask your partner or check it out on screen or in the mirror. Let's play with different leads.

Which Part Leads?

Walk around with the chest leading; with the shoulders leading; with the hips leading; the nose leading; the chin, the knees, the feet. Whichever feels normal or easy is likely to be your own habit.

Leading from the Hip

In the last lesson I got you to lead your partner around the room by the head. This week, lead them again from behind with their eyes closed, but instead of steering them from the head, place your hands on either side of their pelvis. Same rules: when you take your hands off, they stop. Swap it round.

How was that? It's different from guiding someone by the head, isn't it? It's a little more clunky, it feels like a bigger movement, not quite so refined and articulate. However, some prefer to be led by the hips – it feels safer, more held and less flexible, and maybe it's more in their comfort zone, nearer their habitual way of walking. Maybe they are people who lead from the hip!

Check out the National Geographic YouTube video of a cheetah, the fastest animal on the planet, running in slow motion: (youtu.be/_oEA18Y8gM0)[1] It demonstrates how the whole body is organised around the head. The head is still and directed at the prey. Amazing, isn't it?

So let's return to all-fours ourselves. One of the best ways to help us shift our habitual way of walking is to go back to basics and practise crawling.

For the stiff-legged, the sloucher, the bottom-wiggler, the bouncer, the turnout fan, those who lead from the hip and those with uncoordinated limbs, I commend you to crawling. Here we go.

Crawling

From a standing position, take one leg back and lower yourself to one knee, take the other knee back so you are on two knees, bend forward from your newly discovered hip joint and let the hands drop to the floor to support you under the shoulders. Do not brace your arms, and have your hands pointing forward. Make sure the knees are under the hip joints. Find an easy balance so there is more weight on the legs than the arms. Remember not to drop the neck, but keep the length of the spine, going up to the ears and the top of the head, directed towards the wall. Then do it the opposite way so you can experience the difference: brace your arms, have your hands in front of your shoulders and your knees behind your hips so you are more stretched out, and drop your neck. I think you'll find that your spine arches and you're having to use more muscular effort. So take your head back up, so the spine is still extending to the AO joint , move your hands under your shoulders, unbrace your arms and bring your knees under your hip joints. You will find yourself more easily supported.

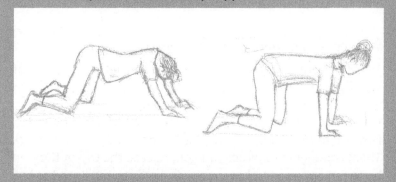

Think of your head leading you as you rock forward and back, spine following the head. Rock forward and back a couple of times and then, as your head comes forward next time, slide one knee forward and let the opposing hand come forward; slide the other knee forward and bring the other hand forward. Continue this movement. It is important to slide the lower leg, to let it caress the floor, otherwise you will be lifting the pelvis up from the lower back. This exercise in crawling is for you to practise not lifting the pelvis as you walk but maintaining the integrity of the head, neck and back, and using the hip, knee and ankle joints easily. Crawl away as long as it is reasonably comfortable; head–spine–knee–hand, head–spine–knee–hand – there's no rush. Then find a chair or the wall and use it to help you crawl upwards into standing and take a walk… Now you may sense how the head is leading and the rest is following; that you feel weirdly coordinated without having to think about it.

It's a really good idea to practise crawling a few steps at least after lying in semi-supine. Being on all-fours is the upside-down version of semi-supine, and it's a great way of taking yourself into movement and the upright.

If crawling isn't your thing – perhaps you have a wrist or knee injury which makes it difficult to work on the floor – here is another experiment for all to play with that will help you explore the crawling motion in an upright position.

Walking on the Spot

Stand in front of a full-length mirror with your feet parallel or slightly turned out, and look to the top of your head. Think of your neck freeing, to allow your head to be released upwards, the back lengthening and widening, and walk on the spot. Notice if there is a displacement going on in the head and torso. Then, continuing to direct yourself, release the top of the shin bone forward so your heel peels off the floor, but keep the ball of your foot in contact with the floor. In other words, you don't want to take the foot entirely off the floor, so the weight can be evenly distributed through both feet. Then take your heel back down on to the floor, and then swap the movement to the other leg. Keep your hands on your hip joints to remind yourself that that's where the leg bones are moving from. It's a way of walking on the spot but not taking the foot off the floor. As the legs are making this movement you are thinking of staying up and centred, so there is as little displacement as possible. When you can manage this relatively easily, take your hands off your hip joints and allow your arms to move in opposition to your knees. As the right knee comes forward, take the left arm forward. The ribs are also moving to accommodate this rotation, as is your spine. Throughout, keep your head still, like the cheetah, looking forward at your reflection. The movement is slow and sustained, and may feel very unnatural. That's okay, it's an exercise to play with, to practise inhibiting the old ways of walking, using the mirror to guide you. A good plan is to ask the reflection in the mirror to do this action, as though you are following it. It's different, isn't it? This way you will be more objective, keep your attention out, relying on your visual sense, not your own internal feelings. If you are working in pairs without a mirror, have one observe and assess the movement, tell your partner if the head and torso are being displaced. And find a mirror to play with during the week as part of the assignments. After playing with this movement for some time, turn around (head leading, of course) and, whilst starting with the rotation, and letting your heel rise as the shin drops forward, walk around without deliberately changing anything. Maybe something has shifted?

Walking is good practice in exploring Alexander's idea that our movement is organised around the head. This seems rational, in that most of our senses are in our head – we see, hear, taste and smell up there, our eyes and ears contribute to our sense of space and balance. Our senses are receiving the stimulus of the environment and we respond to it – just as, when babies, we developed our neural networks in response to the world around us. On a simple level, maybe we hear something, we look towards it and choose whether we want to get closer or run like crazy in the other direction. (Either: 'Oooh, coochy, little kitten...' Or: 'Aargh! Monster spider about to drop on my head!') If the neck is free and the head can turn easily, we will take in more of the world, like meerkats on sentinel duty.

Turning Heads

Take a seat and let's play with some head turning. Remember the AO and AA joints, the most freely movable in the whole spine, right up at the top? When we turn our head, we often tip the head slightly to one side without meaning to. If we are turning to the right, the right ear may get closer to the right shoulder. Does that happen with you? Check it out with a partner or in the mirror. One way of keeping it on the same plane is to think of the opposing eye leading the movement.

Rear-Wheel Drive

As you turn the head to the right, direct the left eye to lead the turn to the right, and as you turn the head back to centre, direct the right eye to lead. Experiment with turning to the other side, too, with this rear-wheel drive. Do you find the head stays more on an even plane? One to practise. If you are visually impaired, experiment by thinking of the opposing ear leading the movement. After all, the organs of balance are right there in the inner ear. The neck muscles are coordinated with the movement of the eyes. Place the flat of your fingers on the top of your neck at the back and, without rotating the head, look from left to right. Can you feel the deep muscles working there? They are anticipating the movement of the head simply from the movement of the eyes.

Unlocking the Eyes and the Head

Here's another great exercise for investigating the eye–head coordination and unlocking its habitual parameters. Using both eyes and head, look as far as you can to the right, clock what you are looking at, then turn back to centre. Now, keeping your head still, let the eyes turn to the right a little way and then let the head follow. Turn back to the centre the same way – eyes first, then the head. Turn again to the right, and this time let the eyes stay looking forward as you turn the head. Then let the eyes join the head. And do the same on the way back to centre – send the head first and then let the eyes follow. Not so easy, that one! Now let the eyes and head turn again together to the right. Clock what you are looking at. Has the head turned a little further? It may have. Experiment with the other side also. Sometimes the other side has already learned from the first, and the difference may not be so pronounced.[2]

The Eyes Have It

Have another walk around, letting the head lead. More fluid? Perhaps it is better to think of the eyes leading, rather than the head. The eyes are leading because we want to look at something, or investigate it. So, walk around deliberately looking at things, taking in the environment; look at the things that interest you. Or maybe there's a sound that draws you? Interesting, isn't it?

We are returning to this whole notion of attention to the outside world. If we are present in a unified field of attention, the relationship of the head, neck and back will change. Instead of being held in a good or bad position the result will be dynamic, balanced, changing from moment to moment. So maybe it is neither the eyes nor the ears leading. Maybe something just catches our attention and we respond, so after all it is the environment or our impulse in response to it that is leading.

The Power of Thought

Since we've circled back to attention and intention – doing something because we want to, not because we ought to, got to, should, must – I want you to experience the power of thought: to give consent or not give consent. And, conveniently, it's to do with head turning. Solo artists: this is one to read thoroughly and then find a friend to play with as part of this week's assignment if you can. It is a really important one to experience.

Giving Consent

As we practised last week, have one person sitting and the other person standing behind, little finger in groove, with the rest of their fingers on their partner's head above the ear. Person Sitting, allow the Person Standing to turn your head very gently as before, so you can look to the right and then to the left. This accomplished, Person Standing is going to try rotating your head again but this time, Person Sitting, do not let them, do not give consent for your head to be turned even a little way. Person Standing, do not try to wrench their head off. You will simply feel unable to move it. It will have locked up with no effort from Person Sitting. Person Sitting, just as a comparison, decide you will give consent again. Person Standing, I bet you suddenly feel that a key has been turned in a lock, as the head moves freely again under your guidance. That's the extraordinary power of thought. It takes no muscular strength or force, just a desire to move or not to move. If you agree to move all of you, all of you will move, as best you can. If you are physically challenged and get around differently – perhaps you use a chair, or sticks or prosthetics – this same premise applies. 'As best you can' is a great phrase, it doesn't mean more than you can, or trying hard to perfect something, it means just what it says on the tin. If you give consent to move, you will move if you are functionally able to. Now swap over, so you both experience the power of thought in both ways.

Taking the Story Out of Your Fist

Make a fist. I expect there's a certain amount of tension in that fist and it's attached to the emotional thought of what we make a fist for – to throw a punch, or defend ourselves. Now let go of the fist: is that a direct action? Or is it simply not doing something? Now let the tips of your fingers touch the palm of your hand and allow the tip of the thumb to rest on your middle finger. I think you may have made a fist again but this time without the habitual tension. It may not be very good for punching, but it is a fist shape nonetheless (and I hope you are not wanting to hit anyone anyway). You are using just the right amount of effort required for now.

Walk This Way

Let's consider your walking habits again. When we were copying and exploring different walks and you stopped leading by the nose, or stopped bouncing, perhaps that was easy because those were not things you usually do. You didn't have to tell yourself to do something different, you simply stopped doing whatever that new way of walking was. Is it possible for you to stop doing your own habit that easily? Have a go.

Walking without Your Habit

If you are now clear about what your own way of walking is, what happens when you just agree not to walk like that? Think of one aspect of your walking: perhaps you hold one of your arms rather stiffly by your side, or pull your head back or sink into your hips, or lead with your chest – just think of one thing you know you do and instruct yourself to let go of it. Walk now without that particular idiosyncrasy. Is it possible? Without saying to yourself, 'I will put my head straight' or 'I will swing my arms' or offering another alternative. Don't 'do' anything different, just don't do whatever that habit is. And if you manage to stop doing that one thing, what happens to the rest of the walking pattern and how does it feel?

Is it enough to just not do the habit? Sometimes we can free ourselves up so that we can walk easily but still be in our habit, and sometimes we can free ourselves up in order to relinquish our habit entirely. Let's add some direction.

Walk with Direction

Add the spatial parameters to your experience of walking. Think of the distance between your head and the ceiling, the space between your back and the wall behind, the space to the left and right of you, whilst also being aware of the space in front that you are walking into. Go walk with those thoughts. Different again?

And then there's *The Travelator*, allowing the space in front to come towards you, allowing the future to come towards you. How's that?

Now change to thinking of Alexander's directions, allowing the neck to be free, to allow the head to go forward and up, and to let the back lengthen and widen, with the knees going forward and away...

Which of all these ways works for you? Maybe they all do.

I hope you are beginning to understand that in Alexander the work is to become aware and experiment with how to change the things you want to change, finding what works for you.

Reverse Up!

Walking Backwards to Walk Forwards

Have a go at walking backwards. How is that? Alarming, maybe, because you can't see where you are going. But once you've got used to that, some of you may notice it feels fairly coordinated and easy. We have no habits of walking backwards (unless you have been trained to do this as a dancer), so as you walk backwards you are walking out of habit and your system is working very happily to balance you. Let's use the technique Alexander used for speaking. Come to a directed state, as best you can, and as you are about to walk forward say, 'No!' to yourself and ask 'Am I free to walk backwards instead?' If you are, then you are free to walk forwards. How is that? Different?

Often we begin our walking by pushing the pelvis forward first. When we walk backwards or prepare to walk backwards, the hip joints release to let the pelvis come back in space, and the top of the torso counterbalances by coming slightly forward.

Not always, of course. If you have learned to tip backwards and tighten the back when walking backwards, then this won't work at all. In this case, experiment instead with thinking that you are about to pick something up. As we go to pick something up, the same new balance starts by freeing the hip joints, sending the pelvis back and the top of the torso slightly further forward. Practise this several times. Remember our habit is there, just with the thought of doing something – the brain has prepared us via the old neural pathways. By giving ourselves another option, the brain is no longer trying to 'get something right' or narrowing its focus, but coming to a wider attention.

How Are You Walking Now?

Once again, observe yourself in the mirror, film yourself or get your partner to copy your walk. Walk without thinking anything in particular. Has something changed just in these first attempts to observe and change how you walk? Then walk again, deliberately choosing different options of thinking – spatial directions, thinking of walking backwards, allowing the world to come to you, just not doing that thing you always do, letting the head turn in response to what you see around you, thinking of your neck freeing and head rising up and leading the movement; remember how the shin bone drops, the heel peels off, and where your hip joint is located. Which works best for you? Are you walking taller, more fluidly, more easily, gracefully? Or just a little differently?

A theatre student who was used to walking in a really cool 'hip-hop' way was told after these experiments that he looked more stiff! He wasn't, of course; he had increased his height and presence. He just wasn't walking as people were used to seeing him walk, and his friend misinterpreted his taller, more effortless minimal gait as stiffness. Here is an example where we can absolutely choose how we want to walk and extend our range, and use our habit if it suits us better. Most of all, remember not to think so much that you start concentrating and cutting off the world like a zombie or – 'Alexandroid' as it's come to be known. That really would look stiff.

Last week your assignments were to think of the head leading as you walked, the way it sits on the top of your spine; to think of the front of the spine occasionally, to practise looking up, opening the jaw, and sending the head up and over to meet the jaw; to look at pictures of the AO and AA joints, the spine, the muscles of the neck and back, to print out pictures and stick them up on the wall, and to use the spatial directions, or Alexander's directions, as you lie in semi-supine for ten to twenty minutes every day. How did your assignments go? Did you manage it all? Did you remember?

We can change in a moment, but we need to keep remembering to change! Not always, of course – it would be impossible to be conscious all the time, but with all the attention exercises you are playing, you are already becoming a little more conscious than you were. When you first become conscious of a habit of mind and body it may initially seem worse, as though you are doing it more. It isn't worse, it's just that you have become more aware of it. So pat yourself on the back – something's changing. And whatever you do, don't try hard! I'm giving you a lot of things to play with, you may not manage them all, or you may have some of your own experiments you want to try out. It's all entirely your choice. Here are the suggestions for this week.

Assignments

- Semi-supine, and after semi-supine, roll over onto all-fours and practise crawling, if only a pace or two, and crawl up the chair or wall to standing.

- Experiments in walking, as we have played with in this lesson.

- Copy the walks of strangers in the street, very surreptitiously – not just for entertainment!

- Practise turning the head with the eye movements.

- Solo artists: find a friend when you can to demonstrate the power of thought.

'I thought about how I could stop taking large strides that were causing my legs to over stretch and my weight to shift from hip to hip in a strange swagger. The teacher suggested I walk backwards and then keep that feeling and thought process as I walked forward. As we walk backwards we tend to take smaller steps and at last my whole body weight felt as though it was distributed evenly throughout my body.' George, drama student

'Whenever I walk, my body is interrelated with the world in which and on which I take my steps. This presupposes some harmony between body and world. We know from physics that the earth rises infinitesimally to meet my step, as any two bodies attract each other. The balance essential in walking is one that is not solely in my body; it can only be understood as a relationship of my body to the ground on which it stands and walks. The earth is there to meet each foot as it falls, and the rhythm of my walking depends on my faith that the earth will be there.' Rollo May[3]

Lesson Five: Eloquence with Elegance

Experiments in sitting and speaking conversationally

Equipment

- A long mirror
- Your recording device
- Chairs
- A watch or clock
- Tennis balls or similar – and space to throw them
- A device with internet access
- Plasticine

'I must neither push my thought nor let it drift. I must simply make an internal gesture of standing back and watching, for it was a state in which my will played policeman to the crowd of my thoughts, its business being to stand there and watch that the road might be kept free for whatever was coming. Why had no one told me that the function of will might be to stand back, to wait and not to push?' Marion Milner[1]

How is the walking? Did you dare to play with copying someone's walk on the street? Review this for yourself, and feel free to share your discoveries with your group or partner. Which way of thinking helped you in exploring your walking pattern – the travelator, the head leading, the crawling or the cross patterning in the mirror, the 'walking backwards' thought, spatial thinking, taking in the outside world – or simply inhibiting one habit? These experiments are ongoing, of course. Whichever way you found helpful, use it!

Mind the Gap!

In this lesson we will look at habits of talking and sitting, and explore further Alexander's notion of inhibition, i.e. stopping the activation of neural pathways from brain to muscle.

How Do You Speak?

If you're in a pair, sit opposite one another. In a group, have two people opposite and one sitting a little distance away and able to observe the pair in profile. If you are working on your own, film yourself *en face* and again in profile. The person designated 'speaker' is going to spend a minute talking about how they got here today, or what they have been doing earlier – anything that occurs to them, really. The one sitting opposite is going to imitate the sitting shape and movements of the speaker. Please note: do not imitate the voice or the lip movements. We are playing with the action, not the sound. The observer will call time and then whisper in the ear of the imitator to coach them on anything they may not have picked up. Get the speaker to continue with the newly coached imitator for a little while longer. Pairs, you will have to do without the coach. And, of course, swap round so everybody gets a go at talking and being observed. Solo artists, film yourself, play it back and jot down what you perceive. Then record yourself again whilst doing the habits deliberately if possible, and play it back to see more clearly what those habits are. And have a laugh at yourself.

This can be an eye-opener. Because we are concentrating on what we are saying, all the various facial twitches, hand movements and foot-tappings that accompany our speaking feel natural, normal – and are quite unconscious. Over the coming week, imagine you're an alien watching earthlings speak to each other: a face that was still will light up and strange movements will occur, all slightly different from each other. Some earthlings will wave their arms about, laugh a lot; sometimes a head will tilt to one side, or the head will move constantly. In this exercise, being an earthling and having instant feedback from your alien partner can be slightly off-putting, and it can take some focus to keep going. Did you find that you were sitting forward or back? Leaning to one side, or using the back of the chair? Were you sitting with your arms and legs crossed, were you slightly collapsed, or sitting bolt upright? How was your tempo? Rushed, slow, thoughtful? You may have been very still and unanimated. This, too, is your habit. How conscious were you of these patterns? Perhaps it is something you are already aware of as we spend more and more time sitting at a screen, and watching ourselves on Zoom? Those facial tics and unheeded mannerisms are blown up tenfold in a close-up on screen and may be entirely inappropriate for your role. Could you change that if your director asked you to? Can you inhibit your reaction to speaking and allow something else to occur?

Our thoughts are very rapid. Our reaction time between receiving a stimulus and reacting to it is a split second.

Passing the Pulse (1)

If you are in a group, hold hands in a circle and have one person squeeze the hand of the person next to them, and that person pass it on to their neighbour until the first person receives the squeeze back again. Time it. Divide the time by the number in the group and you will get an average time. A twenty-third of a second? Have another go and see if you can do it more quickly – send the pulse round the other way, or with your eyes closed – does that make it quicker or slower?

Our perception of time is erratic. 'How can I possibly pause before speaking to change my response? My partner or an audience would get bored waiting for me to speak.' Actually, the audience wouldn't even notice, and it may be that the pause will slow your rate of speech by some milliseconds, making it much easier for the audience to take in what you are saying. The pause in which we can make a choice about how we respond is rather like the TARDIS in *Doctor Who*, bigger on the inside than the outside. The gap between stimulus and our response is bigger on the inside of our experience than is perceived from the outside. Alexander wrote:

> 'My technique is based on inhibition, the inhibition of undesirable, unwanted responses to stimuli, and hence it is primarily a technique for the development of the control of human reaction.'[2]

Hence my taking some time ensuring you become familiar with this. It is the essence of his work.

Passing the Pulse (2)

In the circle again, rather than timing how fast the pulse travels round – and doesn't it seem like an electrical pulse as the squeeze gets passed on? – give yourself the option to change the direction it travels. When someone squeezes your hand, decide whose hand you will squeeze in response – the one whose hand squeezed yours, or your neighbour's on the other side. Now you have a choice. (You may notice in this game that there is a 'short circuit' where two people keep squeezing the others' hand, passing the 'current' back and forth!) You can also choose to slow the pulse by not reacting immediately, but taking your time to choose whose hand you will squeeze. You may find that sometimes the impulse to squeeze affects both hands at once!

We cannot control the outside world, but we can control our reaction to it. We can choose how we respond, and therein lies our power.

Do you remember the childhood game in which you stand opposite someone with hands together, fingers touching, and whoever is leading has to slap the hands of the person opposite before they have a chance to take them away? Similar to 'Knuckles', only the latter is more painful! It's an early game of testing reactions. Feel free to play this in pairs. These days you can surf the internet to find cognitive reactive tests – touch the space bar as soon as you hear this noise, for example – and they are used in the diagnosis of cognitive disorders. Solo artists, check this one out and have a go: playback.fm/audio-reaction-time

Playing Ball

Throw and Catch

Soloists, throw a ball from one hand to the other with a good curving trajectory – no straight-line passing allowed! Throw with both the dominant and the non-dominant hand. If you are in a pair or a group, stand a few feet away from each other and throw the ball between you for a while. As you throw the ball shout 'Stimulus!' and as you catch it, shout 'Reaction!' Discuss.

Within that simple task of throwing and catching are learned habits and emotional responses to the learning. Some of you may have been good at sports and ball games, and love the experience of throwing and catching. Others may have a different story: fearful, as the ball comes towards them, that it will hurt them or that they will drop it and appear stupid. If you bat a balloon to a baby, they may reach out spontaneously towards it but they are not trying to catch it – they haven't learned that skill yet.

Not Catching

Throw the ball again from one hand to the other or to each other, but this time choose not to catch it. Stand there, let the ball come over but stay standing and let it bounce wherever. Or move out of the way if you think it might hit you. But don't catch. Practise this a few times. How does it feel? What happens?

In a group this often inspires a lot of laughter – it seems such a crazy thing to do. Some sporty sorts will find their hand reaching out to the ball despite their best endeavours, and others feel a great sense of relief that they don't have to try catching it at all! You are inhibiting the usual reaction to the stimulus of a ball being thrown, and suddenly there is a creative spirit abroad... Not because you were trying to do something different, but simply by not doing what you usually do. Remember, this is what Alexander did when he thought of speaking and then gave up that intention. It brings us to the creative unknown space, the space without habit. When we lie down in semi-supine and do nothing for ten to twenty minutes, we are practising living in this inhibitory space, not reacting to the phone pinging, or the inner urge to keep busy.

In the end, Alexander did want to speak (he loved acting!), so to inhibit the neural network that associated speaking with excessive tension, he gave himself choices: to speak, not to speak, or to do something else like raise his arm. Here's your choice with the ball.

To Catch or Not to Catch? (1)

Make a choice either to catch the ball or not, or to move out of the way. But don't make the choice until the ball is thrown – do not plan your reaction but simply respond in the moment as the ball comes towards you. Solo artists, as you throw the ball, decide whether to catch it by standing there with your hand ready to receive, to catch it by reaching out, or just drop your hand. Play this for a minute or two.

How was that? Amazing how time slows down as the ball comes towards you and your brain feverishly decides during that time whether to catch or not! After a while you'll find you will make the choice according to how the ball is being thrown; sometimes you will find it seems to be plucked out of the air very easily, as if it were in slow motion, hovering there and waiting for your hand. And if you are throwing the ball from one hand to the other, you will find that, surprisingly, it will sometimes drop into your other hand all by itself. This is the start of learning to juggle, of course – not trying to catch the ball, but learning to throw the ball where you want it to go.[3]

To Catch or Not to Catch? (2)

Play it one more time and, as you throw, shout 'Stimulus!' and, as you catch or don't catch, or move out of the way, shout 'Response!' For in this way we are responding appropriately in the moment, not in a habitual repeated action/reaction.

Stimulus and Response

I've been focusing on the ball coming to your hand as the stimulus. The world constantly throws stimuli at us, and we are consciously or unconsciously responding to them according to our experience and what we pay attention to. Our system is like one big satellite receiver. On a very simple level, suppose we wake in the morning and realise it's a cloudy day outside and raining. How do we respond to that? Immediately feel dull and down because of the weather? If we were going on a picnic it might mean we need to change our plans, or if we were due to spend a day inside studying it might suit us well. We can be pretty good at blaming the outside stimulus for our reaction. A situation may be challenging, but do we have to get anxious or stressed by it? The adrenalin we generate when we are scared is the same adrenalin we get when we are excited – so which is it to be? It's very liberating to separate our response from the stimulus. We cannot change the stimulus but we do have a choice about how we respond to it. 'I'm not listening to the president any more because whatever he says makes me feel angry.' Nothing *makes* you angry. You can choose how you respond and change your action. In 2002 the Dalai Lama and a small group of Western scientists discussed this very thing.[4]

Whilst on the one hand, scientists speak of inhibiting the angry impulse and the resulting action – e.g. not punching someone on the nose but talking to them about the problem – on the other hand, Buddhists aim to make an earlier inhibition to the stimulus, at the very thought of anger; the moment the situation is appraised – e.g. someone has spilt beer over me. So now anger doesn't arise. Neurologically there are three moments of inhibition; one at the appraisal, one at the impulse, one at the moment of action. In Alexander Technique we are exploring all of these, and with diligence we can perhaps find an inhibitory state, a state of grace where we appraise differently. It's not uncommon for the personal friends and family of someone studying Alexander Technique to comment on how much nicer and easier to live with they have become – an added bonus to wanting to change how we balance and move ourselves.

Here's what Tom, one of my acting students, found when applying inhibition to his usual habit of clowning around, switching off and becoming bored:

> 'Romeo and Juliet, the new play that we had just started, was the perfect opportunity to find a solution to the problem. Shakespeare was something I had never done before. Getting frustrated and joking around went hand in hand. So in order to tackle the problem I had to stop getting frustrated. Frustration generally comes from boredom, so I made it my duty to get more involved in the project. I volunteered to get costumes for the play; I offered a whole range of music for the show, and at every opportunity I would throw in new ideas for the scenes I was involved in. I had no time to disengage. I'd still joke around a bit but almost always at the appropriate time... I found that it was becoming easier to listen and learn rather than mess around... it was incredible to notice just how much resisting the urge to disrupt was improving me as an actor. I felt a new-found confidence in performing as I wasn't shying away behind a stream of jokes... Our

director commented on my high level of professionalism and creativity in rehearsal... As for the clown in me, he's still there as big as ever, but I've learned to control him more effectively.'

Apart from responding to a stimulus outside ourselves, we also respond to a stimulus within – we have intentions and desires to take action. In our game with the balls, it is a desire to throw. Alexander had a desire to speak. An intention. So let's use inhibition to play with this internal stimulus, to help us out of habit.

To Throw or Not to Throw?

In pairs again or on your own, have the ball in your hand and a desire to throw. As you begin the movement, take note of all that preparation of muscle, as though you and the arm are filling up with the thought of throwing. In that moment, choose not to throw and, as you sense the release of that thought in the muscle itself, throw. In this way the throw is one of release, not one of habit or contraction or trying. A new neural pathway. As the ball is thrown, choose again whether to catch the ball or not. Play this a number of times. Then, if you are working in a group, have half of you watch the other half do the exercise for a while and then swap round. If you are working in a pair or solo, film yourself and watch it back.

What do you notice? I bet you find it bizarrely riveting. Who would think throwing and catching a ball could be so dramatically entertaining? It's not the action but the thought that is so interesting. You are watching someone thinking and making a decision. You don't know if the ball is going to be thrown, or when/whether it will be caught or left to drop. The unknown creative space. Living in the moment outside of habit, outside of the prescriptive text, outside of the predictable. And what's one of the greatest attributes of a fine actor?

Here's another great game to explore inhibition, the key to change.

The Hot Seat

Solo artists, imagine someone you don't know is in front of you and you have permission to ask them ten or more questions. Write these questions down on separate pieces of paper, or you could film yourself asking them. Come back to this book once you've done that, and I'll have more instructions later in this section.

Pairs – you are Horse and Carriage. Sit opposite each other, or look to each other on screen during your Zoom call. Carriage ask Horse a question – whatever randomly comes into your mind. Maybe the question will come because of something you notice about your partner, or maybe it's something you've always wanted to know and been afraid to ask! Horse, decide in the moment, according to the question asked, how you will respond. You have three choices: to answer truthfully, untruthfully, or not at all. If you don't answer, Carriage will get the idea and ask you another question. When you have played this for at least ten questions, swap it round.

Group – sit in a circle. Have someone in 'the hot seat'. They look at someone else in the circle, and in that moment and not before (resist or inhibit the need to plan ahead), the person being looked at thinks of a question they want to ask. Again, it may be stimulated by the person, or perhaps by a question that's been asked before. If nothing comes to mind, wait until it does. There's no hurry. When the question arrives, the person in the hot seat also doesn't have to answer immediately but has time to make the choice whether to answer truthfully, untruthfully, or not at all. If the person doesn't want to answer, they will look to someone else, and the game continues until at least ten questions have been asked. It can go on for as long as you like, but after a while give someone else a go in the hot seat.

Solo artists – randomly select a question from those you wrote down earlier and play this same game, answering truthfully, untruthfully, or not at all. I suggest you speak out loud, as it makes clear the action from the thought. If you have recorded your questions and are using a screen, use the pause button to ensure you can answer – or not answer – in your own time! Go through all your questions.

Please note: in all cases please choose to experience *all three options*. There is an underlying cultural agreement that we should answer truthfully, and it is also considered rude not to reply. For the purposes of this game, these social customs are eliminated. Enjoy!

The Art of Inhibition

We often imagine that the role of the hot seat will be difficult or intimidating, but it is the easiest role in the world – you are in charge, you are in control; it's up to you whether you tell the group who you are having sex with, where you got your blue top from, or what films you enjoy. You are beginning to experience Alexander's 'Constructive Conscious Control of the Individual'.[5] And I can tell you, it's great fun making up some porkies. I was once asked what I did for a living and I replied 'a car mechanic'. It led to some very interesting spin-off questions, which I also lied my way through and thus created a whole new reality for myself. Of course this is not an encouragement to lie or be rude, but simply to start giving yourself a choice. That's the empowerment. Rather than answering an email or text right away, maybe it's okay to pause and wait for a while. Or write it, but don't send it until the next morning. Who's in the hot-seat anyway? The person asking a question also often feels pressure to think of something to ask – how powerful it is to pause and wait until a question comes to mind, keep the hot-seat person waiting. Both of you are using the inhibitory pause.

So, we've been addressing how we can change some of our habitual reactions to speaking by pausing, by inhibiting our reaction to a stimulus – speaking not 'on voice' but how we speak conversationally, how we express ourselves in day-to-day life. You see, Alexander discovered that what he was doing in public speaking was present in his normal speech, too, but as it wasn't so pronounced, he could get away with it.

The habit

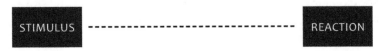

Alexander's technique to stop the habit, inhibiting reaction to stimulus

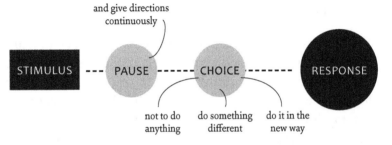

Sitting Pretty

In the opening exercise and this last one, you were sitting. And your partner at the beginning imitated the way you sat: leaning back into the chair, crouched forward, feet together, legs splayed apart – all habitual stuff. So to improve your voice, we need to look at the whole pattern of use. Let's consider a useful way of sitting that is neutral, out of habit and easy. (This is also jolly useful to combat the effects of spending more time sitting at a computer screen, which is often sucking us into its virtual reality and pulling us out of shape!)

One way is to check our body map again. We know where the head meets the spine at the atlanto-occipital joint; where the spine begins and ends; that the support of the spine is in the front; and the location of the hip joint is at the side of the pelvis where the femur inserts, and is your halfway point. Essential knowledge for easy walking. For easy sitting, let's check out the pelvis. Look it up online and you will see it three-dimensionally in all its glory. Meanwhile, here's an illustration.

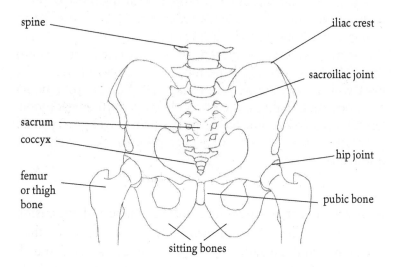

You will notice that it is made up of two bones that attach to the spine at the sacrum and are jointed together at the pubic bone with cartilage. This is not a freely movable joint but fixed – although during pregnancy the joint softens to allow the baby to come out. This is also true of the connection to the spine at the sacrum. The spine is lashed to the pelvis with ligament at the sacroiliac joints, and though the joint is very firm, there is also a little 'give' in it. Sometimes, however (and not just in pregnancy), these joints will be dislodged and need a spine specialist to click them back into place. This can sometimes be due to our pressurising the spine, pushing it down as we pull the head back and down. (In the flexible, miniature model skeleton I use when teaching to demonstrate this compression of the spine, it is always the wire around its sacroiliac joints that 'gives' and needs to be repaired.)

The Plasticine Pelvis

Take a piece of plasticine or modelling clay and, using the pictures here and on the internet for guidance, construct a tiny pelvis. It's a great way of discovering its extraordinary shape and getting to know it better. I would suggest modelling one side at a time and sticking them together at the pubic bone. It really is two side bones, slightly twisted and joined. The sitting bones, pubic bone and iliac crest are all part of the same bone; the names just refer to different areas. (The iliac crest is where the waist begins and is often mistaken for part of the 'waist joint' which, as we know, doesn't exist.) Remember your model does not have to be perfect. No gold stars for the best model here. You can play some music and suck on a sweetie as you do it – it's just a way of learning through play. You could keep it as a souvenir.

Now you are better acquainted with the shape and dimension of the pelvis, feel it in your own body. It's a little firmer than plasticine! Find the outline of the pelvis at the back, top and all the way down the front. You will notice that there is very little space between the floating ribs and the top of the pelvis at the back. The top of the pelvis is there for muscle attachment, not for support. The thickest areas of your pelvis are in the sockets of your hip joint and in the sitting bones – these are the main places of support.

Are You on Your Rocker?

Sit on your hands for a moment, palm up, and rock forward and back – that's the sitting bones working for you. They are like the rockers on a rocking chair, coming towards each other at the front until they become the pubic bone. Take your hands away and have your feet in front of you, directly below your knees. Now, letting your head lead and not bending at the waist, do circles on your sitting bones by tipping your torso forward, to the right, to the back and to the left, and then circle back the other way. You will notice it is easier somehow to tip forward – the legs are out there in front to support you. So often we imagine our legs have nothing to do with sitting, but have to be got rid of, tucked away under the seat or held tight, knees together. But just for a moment imagine you were trying to balance on the sitting bones and your legs had disappeared – your stability would be gone in an instant. So let the feet stay under your knees for the moment.

Losing the Arch

Now sit there for a moment with your arms held out in front, elbows released and shoulder-width apart. You are in the same crawling shape that we used for your walking coordination in the last lesson; the same shape we use when lying down in semi-supine. We usually sit with our hands in front, rarely behind us, often moving them in front of us to manipulate a fork, a keyboard or a musical instrument. As you take your arms up in front of you, what happens to your waist and lower back? Do you find yourself arching your lower back again? When we take our arms up in front, we often counteract their weight by pulling our chest up and back and arching the lower back. Maybe, instead, see if you can counteract the weight by lengthening the back, tipping slightly forward and thinking into the sitting bones and feet. Check it out in your pairs, or on your filming device. Interesting, isn't it, how we balance ourselves even in sitting? We don't ever have to be plonked down!

The sitting bones are much closer together than we think. After all, a bicycle saddle is not very wide. Don't feel this out on a partner – it's too intimate! – but trace the sitting bones on the inside between your own legs and out to the pubic bone. Got it now? Just knowing this might make it easier to use them for sitting. If you are on a chair that scoops you back, like a bucket seat, find the edge or even sit astride the corner so you can use the sitting bones. Sometimes sitting astride a chair, facing the back, can be an immense help: the legs will be wider apart than usual, the arms can rest easily on the back, and the crutch is decorously protected by the back of the chair.

Here's a picture of the pelvis from the side.

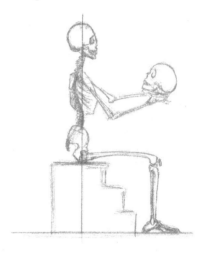

You will see that there is some distance between the coccyx at the end of the spine and the sitting bones at the end of the pelvis. We often sit on the back of the sitting bones, which tips the pelvis back, collapses the spine and puts support through the coccyx.

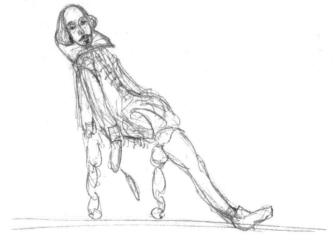

We get away with this because we are often on 'comfy' chairs that cushion the coccyx. Or we are sitting in chairs designed more for stacking than sitting and support us in this poor use. When we sit like this, the head is also unbalanced and the spine is being compressed from both ends. Not a good idea for general practice. We are designed to use our sitting bones for sitting. Sometimes, if we are playing a 'stuck-up' part, like Cecily or Algernon in *The Importance of Being Earnest*, we will again hoick our chest up and tighten our lower back, pushing the lumbar spine forward to find the front of the sitting bones. All very tiring and, because the lower ribs are pushed forward and the diaphragm compromised, it interferes with our breathing. Not good for an actor who needs the breath to flow easily. Also, attempting to hold ourselves up in this way often creates pain in the lower back. Nor will it solve the problem for very long, for we cannot maintain this struggle against gravity – gravity will always win – and after a while we will collapse down again.

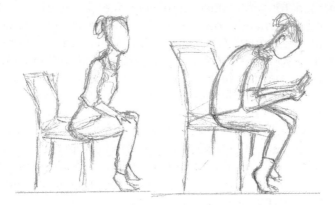

Sometimes we have got into the habit of collapsing in a hunched or semi-foetal position by copying our elders. Sometimes it was because we were simply not wanting to be there. And then someone said 'Sit up straight!' So we did our best by putting on a smile and the braced holding pattern to please the Authority, though our heart was still sorrowful, and not whole heartedly wanting to be where we were, battling our desires as well as gravity. Later, as adolescents, it was perhaps cool to stay down like that, to fit in with the general pattern of use of our classmates. And those school chairs weren't a great help.

So, how can we achieve this new balance in sitting that will both be easy to maintain and allow us to be wholehearted again? Knowing where our sitting bones are will help, for sure, and remember that you want the line of gravity to come down through the front of your spine, the supporting area of spine. When we pull our chest up, the line of gravity is going down the back of the spine. So here's my favourite solution, a movement that happens by attending to the outside world again:

Going Down to Come Up

Allow yourself to be in a nice collapsed position on the chair. Rock forward on your sitting bones until you are almost crouched forward. Make sure your feet are easily on the ground underneath your knee joint, then allow your eyes to look up and around. Allow your head to follow, and your spine to follow your head. You will find yourself sitting up without bracing. It may not feel very upright because it's so easy, and you may feel crumpled, or tipped forward, so do check it out in the mirror or on-screen. I would practise this movement. It's the movement that counts: staying in a balanced, movable, flexible place, not getting into the 'right' position that's held, rigid, fixed and requires effort to maintain. When sitting like this, you may find that a lot of your conversational mannerisms will become redundant and just stop.

Clothes also influence our sitting. If I'm wearing a short skirt, I am not going to sit with my legs wide apart, for obvious reasons! But if we continue to bring our knees tightly together in a holding pattern even when not wearing a short skirt, then we are creating a habit using unnecessary tension. So when it's appropriate, we can let that pattern go. That does not mean when wearing trousers we have an excuse to sit on our coccyx with legs sprawled out in front of us, collapsing! Best not do that either. If a character needs to be in that shape, fair enough. But for you, as a centred, balanced, talented actor, it's important to find an easy, relaxed way of sitting that is coordinated, effortless and not switched off. Use the back of a chair if you like – you don't want to look perched all the time. Also, it can be tiring at first, and not always so easy to find the balanced place just on the sitting bones. But don't collapse back. Keep the torso long, as it is resting. So often we lean back into the centre of the chair back and drop our chest. Remember, your spine continues up to your ears. Keep the spine easily long. And perhaps take the sitting bones to the back of the chair, so there is not so much of a backward angle. Apparently, Alexander would often use his cigar box to support the centre of his back on the back of the chair. Inhibit your desire to collapse when resting on a chair. So there.

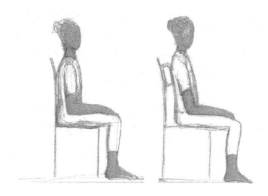

Speaking without Your Habits

Now let's go back to the first exercise in speaking conversationally. Go back to the same pairs or threes. Solo traveller, film yourself again. This time agree to inhibit all your talking habits. Allow yourself to sit quietly and easily in the chair and speak conversationally again, but without the usual pattern of how you sit or nod your head, or whatever it is you do to yourself as you speak. If you are one of those that sits extremely rigidly it may be that you give yourself the freedom to release and move more. Maybe this time you could do a monologue on your favourite films. What was the last one you saw, and what was the first one? Just have a go, even if you feel like a zombie or a formal Victorian – it's just an experiment. Is it possible for you to still express yourself even though you are not moving as usual? The one sitting opposite will still be mirroring you, so you will see a reflection of how you look. What else could you use in your thinking to help with this? Yes, spatial directions, taking in the bigger picture, pausing and making different choices. And feedback from your partners: has something changed? What does it look like? What does it feel like? How likely are you to play with this whilst having a chat with a friend in the coffee shop or on Zoom?

Remember, it's your choice. Suddenly even a casual chat can become part of your training as an actor. Something interesting happens, too, when we are in a group of people we like. We start to copy body shapes; we come into rapport with them. Well, why not take note of that and, next time, see if you can call the shots. Get them to come into your Alexander shape – not by talking about it, just by subtly and discreetly choosing to sit differently, responding in the moment. Maybe they will change shape along with you.

Assignments

- Keep playing with your way of walking.

- Semi-supine. For a change, find a wall to place your feet on, rather than the floor. This is the sitting shape, were you to be suddenly flipped up through ninety degrees.

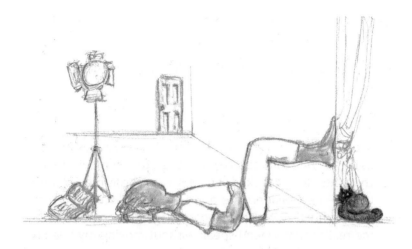

- Practise thinking of your use patterns as you speak socially to friends, and see if you can't change your use and quietly influence those around you as they come into rapport.

- Pause before speaking sometimes.

- Pause before answering your phone. With hands free you don't have to scrunch your shoulder up to hold the phone. If you are using your hand, are you dropping your neck to speak and listen, or are you able to bring the phone to your mouth? Can you be aware of the space around you, even though you are speaking to someone in a different environment? Are you using hand gesticulation, even though you cannot be seen?

- Play with your habits of sitting. Remember not to rush to 'good position', but inhibit your reaction to the stimulus and instead pause, move freely on the sitting bones and look around you, so that you are balancing again. If you find you are in a collapsed state, go further into it; it will start you moving and you can change the movement into tipping forward on your sitting bones, bringing your gaze up, your head following, your spine following the head. You will be unfolding yourself, coming back up into the world, being where you want to be wholeheartedly.

- Prepare or remind yourself of a short monologue to work on next week.

'I know that I move my head a lot when I'm speaking. It's as if I feel that my voice is not enough to communicate my thoughts alone. I looked at people who hardly moved their heads – newsreaders are good at this. I discovered that it looks normal, which was encouraging because it made me realise that when I speak without moving my head it looks normal, even though it feels weird to me! I began to practise saying my lines whilst lying in semi-supine so that I could feel when I lifted my head to speak and choose not to do it. I feel that gradually my habit is changing.' Jennifer, drama student

'She bent her finger and straightened it. The mystery was in the instant before it moved, the dividing moment between moving and not moving, when her intention took effect. It was like a wave breaking. If she could only find herself at the crest, she thought, she might find the secret of herself, that part of her that was really in charge.' Ian McEwan, Atonement[6]

Lesson Six:
The Tottering
Biped Speaks!

Experiments in standing and speaking publicly

Equipment

- Your recording device
- The audio recording of standing meditations, plus speakers or headphones so all can hear easily
- A full-length mirror
- Your logbook
- Balls
- A bean bag or bag of unfrozen peas
- A prepared monologue
- Space to play

'How surely gravity's law,
strong as an ocean current,
takes hold of even the strongest thing
and pulls it towards the heart of the world.'

Rainer Maria Rilke[1]

As you are reading this, are you sitting gracefully? And this week have you been speaking easily, calmly, excitedly, eliminating by choice all unnecessary effort and gesticulations? No? Maybe not, but I hope you've been practising and making your own discoveries along the way. Another thought I had about the pelvis: it is like a three-dimensional bony arch. Any arch has a wedge-shaped keystone in the middle – ours is the sacrum, the wedge at the bottom of the spine. The support from the planet comes up through the feet, the legs and the hip joints or sitting bones, up through the inner rim of the pelvis, up the sacrum and the front of the spine. More of that support later in this lesson.

Did you have a go at influencing others' use simply by changing yours as you chatted? How were the experiments with the phone? How are those lovely sitting bones? Did you enjoy this other way of lying in semi-supine, taking on the crawling/sitting shape, your feet propped against the wall? Check through your logbook (if you are keeping one) to reflect, or share your experiences with your study partner or group.

Stand and Deliver!

Now let's up the ante. Time to see what you get up to whilst you are performing.

Your Habits in Performance

Soloists, film yourself doing a monologue you know well – an audition speech or something you are currently working on. If you are in a pair, act out your speech in front of the other. If you're in a group, try this in threes again – one speaking, two observing. Observers, give feedback on what physical things you see happening to the speaker as they perform. This is not feedback on acting skills: it is a given that you are all wonderful as actors and perform well. But is the speaker standing stiff as a board, are they moving a lot, do they favour one side, do they tighten their legs, do they narrow their attention to a spot in the distance, lean forward to you as the audience, tip their face back, thrust their neck forward, stand with their legs braced, are they windmilling their arms? Whatever you see, when they have finished let them know what you observed. Solo artists, after watching yourselves back on film, jot all these things down. Are they the same things you noticed in that first lesson, when you spoke the first couple of lines of a piece of text on film? Is it possible for the piece to be done again, and for the speaker to take the direction and stop doing those things? Remind yourself of all the ways that might help – thinking spatially, widening the vision, inhibiting the first reaction to speaking. Swap round so you all get a turn at acting in front of your peers and taking some direction regarding your use. Consider if this is something you were aware of and experiment with changing it. One response is perhaps that it doesn't feel right not to do it in that way; that the tensions, movements and balance, although habitual, feel right for that character at that point in the play. If that's the case, mark the piece – don't 'act' it out, but speak the text in a neutral manner and for the time being focus on the use. We are working on Alexander's technique. You can always return to your old way, or add the inner truth later if necessary. This is just an experiment. Play with it and find out. Maybe your beliefs will change...

Sometimes it will feel very wrong – a faulty sensory perception – but the result can be astonishingly powerful. We stop 'doing' and find a genuine connection to the text. One powerful young actor was using so much tension in the passion of the character she played that she was pushing her head forward and visibly straining her neck. 'But if I don't give it my all, it will be untruthful!' she remonstrated with me. But when she lost her voice and couldn't perform, truth was neither here nor there. A good lesson to learn is that, as actors, we need technique so we can play the inner truth eloquently and effortlessly.

Interesting, isn't it? What we think we are doing may not be so, and we may be doing a load of other stuff we had no idea about.

Time for a game. Let's revise the catching and throwing game.

Throw a Question, Catch an Answer

Have a ball in one hand and throw it to the other, calling out 'Stimulus!' when you throw and 'Response!' when you catch – or when you don't; it's your choice.

Or throw and catch in a pair. Now think that extra thought during the activity: of the space above, behind, on either side; a panoramic vision of what's in front, and a sense of the ground under your feet… Maybe that thinking is there anyway, but if not, use it consciously this time. Practise this as you throw and catch for a while longer. Pause. This time, instead of shouting 'Stimulus!', shout out a random question to your hand or partner. If the hand or partner catches the ball, they have to answer the question before throwing the ball back with another question. If the ball is not caught, then there is no reply – the ball is picked up and another question shouted out as the ball is thrown back. Remember, there is no hurry. It may take time to think of a question and to answer. Can you keep the spatial awareness going all the time? Have fun!

The next game uses inhibition to help you improvise. I have seen improvisation where the actors were so nervous about leaving space and time for thought that they filled the gaps with hysterical swearing. This exercise can be as slow and thoughtful as you like, and it makes any necessary swearing more poignant.

To Answer or Not to Answer? An Improvisation

Lose the balls and stand in the same pairs, Egg and Bacon. Stand consciously, spatially aware, same distance as before. You are partners living together. Egg has come home very late. Bacon starts the conversation with 'Where have you been?' Egg can choose to answer or not to answer. If Egg does not answer, then Bacon asks another question and continues until Egg answers. Egg then asks a question of Bacon which will be a stimulus for Bacon to choose whether to answer or not. If Bacon answers, Bacon also must follow it with a question. Keep this going for a few minutes, then swap roles. If you're in a group, do the initial practice all together and then have half the group watch the other half do the exercise and then swap it around. Soloists, you take both parts. Look to your right (remember how the head turns at the top of the spine!) to your imaginary partner and ask the question 'Where have you been?' Make a choice to turn your head to the left or keep it turned to the right. If you turn to the left, you reply to the question and then ask a question of the interrogator. The initial interrogator then decides whether to answer or not, and on it goes. It will generally be the desire to answer or not that dictates the head movement, but you could play it the other way round, by choosing in the moment whether to turn the head or keep it still, with the consequence that you have to speak or not. Feel free to record this and play it back if it helps. Pairs and groups, please note or share what you discover. Perhaps it's exciting, powerful, thoughtful, humorous dialogue spoken by people making conscious choices and taking their space.

Proprioception

You've been practising conscious thinking whilst standing all this time, and implicitly practising balancing. When we sit we have six legs to help our balance – our own legs and the four legs of the chair. When we stand we are a 'tottering biped'[2], a two-legged creature constantly about to fall and, below consciousness, setting off little micro-movements that constantly adjust to give us our stability. What is organising our balance? The vestibular system in our inner ear, our visual system and our proprioception. Proprioception is known as the sixth sense, the sense of our self – the juxtaposition of body parts and effort in movement and equilibrium. It's our sense of belonging – that your leg belongs to you and nobody else. In *The Man Who Mistook His Wife for a Hat*, Oliver Sacks tells the story of a patient who woke alone in hospital after a stroke and felt a stranger's leg in his bed. He hurled the leg out of bed – only to find himself on the floor. The leg, of course, was his own: his proprioception had been damaged by the stroke.[3] Challenge your balance systems for a moment by standing on one leg. Now close your eyes. I bet you could sense your proprioception working, the parts of you wobbling about trying to balance you without the help of your vision. Not so easy to balance. I understand that, when autopilot is set on a jumbo jet, the plane is constantly going off-course. Fortunately, this activates the guidance system that puts the plane back on course. That's like us! However, we often try to hold ourselves up, stopping this healthy movement by fixing and using muscular effort to jam one part of us whilst the other part collapses, and then switching over. You will have experienced this if your tendency has been to stand with your weight on one leg and then when that gets tired, swapping to the other leg. When we stiffen our leg joints we receive little information about balance as nothing is moving. We get the information about effort – it's beginning to hurt – so we shift positions to relieve the pressure. When we are balancing well, there is no effort.

We also use information about the outside world as a reference point for our balance – visually, as we have discovered, but also from what we are in touch with. When we touch someone we are using a sense of them received through our fingertips to balance with. It doesn't mean we are leaning into them, not at all. Both partners are adjusting to each other's balance. You may have experienced this particularly if you were dancing with someone.

Exploring the Foot

Our feet have proprioceptors in the joints and are in touch with the ground most of the time. Take your shoes and socks off and have a good look at your feet. There are twenty-six bones in the foot, one less than in the hand. The length of your foot is the same as your forearm: the distance between the wrist and the elbow. Measure it and see. We never perceive it like that because when we look at our feet it's often at a distance, and anyway we only see the front of the foot. We rarely see the heel unless, like now, you are inspecting it.

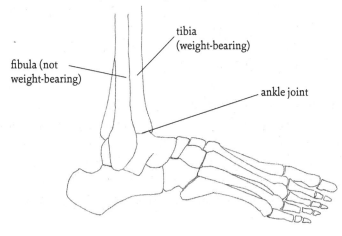

Find a photo of a foot on the internet as well and you will see more clearly that the bones are curved. Arches are a strong structure. The foot has to be supportive, as well as very flexible. The arches of the foot act as shock absorbers, in a similar way to the curves of the spine. There is 'give' in them. They are created by the structure of the bones and supported by ligaments and tendons. We have the longitudinal arches and medial arches and, depending how they are classified and named, we can have three or four. The metatarsal arch that goes across the front of the foot is the one that 'gives' if you squeeze your foot with your fingers. Do that now, have a squeeze of your foot – feels good, doesn't it? This metatarsal arch is very important as support and in giving us the spring in our step for running and dancing. Another line of support I like to think of is the bony connection between the ball of the foot and the heel. The heel is not centred in the back of the foot, by the way; it sits more to the outside. Feel that with your hands.

Thinking on Your Feet

Stand up and think of that diagonal arch between the ball of your foot and the heel. Think also of the connection between the area below your little toe and the heel. Think of the arch across the front of your foot. Lean forward gently from the ankles and, just as we did in the last lesson on the sitting bones – keeping yourself thinking up, legs straight, torso not collapsing or using the 'waist joint', head leading – sway to the right and onto the back of your foot, to the left and onto the front of the foot. Do this a few times and then circle the other way. Look at yourself in the mirror as you do this, or watch another in a group or pair. This is a very useful movement if you ever have to pretend you are drunk or on board a ship.

The circling in that exercise is happening courtesy of your ankle joint. Look at the drawing again and feel your own ankle bones.

They are the end of your tibia and fibula, the bones of your lower leg. Together they, too, form an arch, a saddle that fits over the talus bone. This is the ankle joint. The fibula finishes lower down on the outside of your foot and is not supportive on its own. If you trace a line from the fibula on the outside to the end of the tibia on the inside of your ankle, you will feel the curve of the ankle joint. The talus bone of the foot sits on top of the heel bone or calcaneus, to use its formal name. Between the bones, as in all joints, there is synovial fluid within the capsule of the joint, so you have two cushions of fluid between your leg and the heel.

Feeling the Feet

Stand again, and think about that cushioning support you have in the ankle joint. If you are in a pair or a group, kneel in front of your partner and place your hands over the top of their foot. Don't push into the foot, just let your hands rest there and ask your partner to sway in circles again. You will feel all the bones moving, coordinating and adjusting as they change their balance. Ask them to be still and you may still feel tiny little movements and adjustments. Ask them to take their arms up in front, then above the head and down again. You will feel how the feet are adjusting themselves as necessary to help them balance. Please swap this around. Solo artists, for this exercise you need to find someone to experiment with in the next week, if you can, so you too can feel the movement and have your own feet warmed by someone's hands. Discuss this. What did you experience? It can be very grounding to have someone place their hands on your feet. For others it can be unnerving. If you are squeamish about having someone touch your feet, maybe place a bag of unfrozen peas or a bean bag on them, something heavy that gives and will take the shape of your foot, just to ground you and direct your attention there for a moment or two. (This could also be helpful to those working solo.)

In pairs again, this time whilst kneeling, place the sides of your hands on the outside of your standing partner's foot, cupping your fingers gently round the heel. You who are standing, just be still and think of that connection between the ball of the foot and the heel. And lastly, you who are kneeling, just place the tips of your first two fingers at the front of your partner's ankle joint, either side of the main ligament there, and imagine the fingers directed diagonally down through the joint to the heel behind and below. Sometimes this leads to a curious sensation of the joint opening and freeing, finding a space within itself. Discuss and swap over.

So far we've been paying attention to the feet, the end of us that interfaces with the earth, and to changing or enhancing our body map, which, in turn, can change how we stand. Something else to remember is how big the feet are: the distance between your wrist and the inside of your elbow is about the length of your foot. Imagine them as great clown feet below. We so often hide our feet, imagining them to be solid chunks at the end of our legs – 'plates of meat', as they are called in Cockney rhyming slang. But feet are pliable, responsive and strong – fabulous engineering! We can abuse them terribly, squeezing them into tight-fitting shoes, pointed and with heels, and yet, amazingly, we can still – just about – balance. Bear in mind that babies don't need shoes to get around. There are huge cultural and social habits around footwear. Shoes are there both to protect our feet, and sometimes to make outrageous decorative statements! As actors, you will sometimes need to balance yourself in unusual footwear – remember that men, too, wore fashionable heels in various periods of our history. We can learn to do that with the least effort and pressure on our tootsies, although I wouldn't recommend such footwear as a regular thing. The choice, as always, is yours.

Footsure

Which part of the foot do you tend to favour for your balance? A lot of us stand more on the front of the foot. If you have been in a jazz class, preparing for a Bob Fosse routine, your teacher will no doubt have asked for this, to show you are 'centred' and ready to go. Runners, after they have found their mark at the start of the race, 'get set' on their toes. Society often demands that we keep 'on our toes'. However, life is not always a race or an emergency, and our easy centre does not require this balance.

Balance Yourself Up

Position yourself in front of a mirror and deliberately stand more on the front of your foot. This tends to take the pelvis forward and is often the pose we adopt if someone says, 'Stand up straight!' You will notice, too, that the legs tend to brace themselves and the front of our torso overextend. What's happening up at the top end? Are you dropping your neck forward, or are you tipping your head back? Now watch the top of your head in the mirror. Gently change your balance so that you are putting your weight more on your heel and take the pelvis back underneath you, unbracing the legs. When I say 'take the pelvis back', I don't mean that you tuck the pelvis in or tilt it, but simply imagine it as the end of the long pendulum that is your spine, swinging back from the top of your neck. Bracing the legs often includes tightening the bum, and you may have learned to tuck it under or stick it out. Just let it go, undo any holding in the pelvic area and let it all hang out! Although the line of gravity ideally drops through the ankle joint, I suggest you think of coming back more on the heel, so that you balance further back than you are used to. The line of gravity will adjust to the ankle joint more easily that way. Play with 'penguin feet', lifting the toes off the floor and flapping them so you know there is no support in the front. Pairs, one of you change your balance whilst the other observes the top of your head; and swap. Groups, have one half of the group change the balance whilst the other half observes; and swap. It is quite stunning to see a whole line of people in a group grow by an inch or two!

When we stand on the front of the foot, hips forward, the top of us tends to pull back in counterbalance, creating a curve, a banana shape, which diminishes our height. When we shift our balance by bringing our pelvis back in space and find our support more through the back of the foot, we get taller.

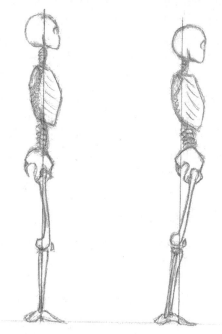

There is also a false belief that, in order for a limb to be at its longest, we need to lock the joints.

Unlocking the Limbs

Face the wall and, with a straight arm held horizontally, place your fingertips on the wall. Gently release the elbow, and you will find you are still touching the wall. You can also do this in a pair, reaching out to your partner's shoulder rather than a wall.

There is more length in the muscles of the limb if you are not tightening or bracing. Again, stand in front of someone who is observing the top of your head, or stand in front of a mirror. With braced legs, gently release the knees forward a little. See how far you can release them before you visibly start to lose height. It's quite a way, isn't it?

So our system is having to work much harder to hold ourselves down in this shortening banana shape. But very easy to change, when we remember. 'There's the rub,' as Hamlet would say. We need to be conscious in order to change. Play again with standing more on the front of the foot and then come back and up as you find the balance more through the back of the foot, and unbrace the legs. So you never have to 'stand up straight' again. Unless you want to, of course, or are playing a character who stands like that. (And even that can be 'cheated' and made easier to maintain. But more of that later...)

Using the Forces of Nature

You will notice that in exploring both sitting and standing I have not used the term 'posture', which suggests a 'good' or 'bad' holding pattern. I prefer the term balance, or poise, or shape, as these indicate already that we are in flux and movement, responding to the forces and stimuli around us without judging anything as 'good' or 'bad'. I advise certain different balances for you as actors because you need to be flexible and adaptable without using vast amounts of unnecessary muscular strength. What natural forces are we responding to? There are four in the universe as currently defined by the laws of physics: gravity, electromagnetism, the weak interaction and the strong interaction. I'm sure Professor Brian Cox could explain all this far better than me, so let us just stick to gravity – and something we know experientially, which is that whilst gravity ensures we are sticking to the surface of the planet and not floating off, we do not sink through to the centre of the earth. The gravitational force of the earth pulling us downward is countered by an equal upward reaction or contact force that stops that. We often forget that one. As we pay attention to the upthrust from our planet, we can change our experience of standing. Here are two standing meditations that may help.

Listen to the audio recordings on standing and try them out. (www.alexanderpen.co.uk/about-the-alexander-technique/alexander-meditations/)

Finding the Marionette Within

In a group or pair you can also read the guidance out to each other before swapping around so everyone gets a turn. Use each ellipsis as a pause, time to allow those standing to consider each instruction:

'Let's pay attention to the gravitational force that is connecting us to the earth below, lengthening us. As you stand there, supported more to the back of the foot, knees releasing, become aware of the space above you, the space behind you, the space on either side of you, and the space in front of you... and now become aware of the balance of the head on the spine, how the face is dropping down, sending the back of the head up... become aware of the spine hanging from the head... each vertebra of the spine hanging from the one above it... the breastbone hanging from the side and back of the head... the collarbones hanging from the breastbone... the shoulder blades from the collarbones... Become aware of the upper arm hanging from the shoulder blade... the lower arm hanging from the upper arm... the hands hanging from the wrists... Become aware of how each rib is hanging from the one above it and from the spine and from the breastbone... Become aware of the pelvis hanging from the ribs and from the spine... the upper leg hanging from the pelvis... the lower leg hanging from the upper leg... the foot dropping out of the ankle and spreading onto the surface of the earth. And having thought through this suspension system, allowing everything to hang down from the head, like a well-strung marionette, take a little walk around.'

How does that feel? Note your experience of it, or talk to a partner about it and swap roles if necessary. It can help stop the habit of trying to hold yourself up from the planet and lead you to a new experience. It can help 'ground' you.

The Up Direction

Now let's get you to think of the other direction, the opposing force: the upthrust of the earth. Listen to the audio recording 'The Up Direction'. If you are flying solo, use the headphones. Pairs and groups, find a speaker so you can all hear the recording. A group could also choose one person to read out the instructions, providing you swap them so they too have that experience. To make it even more powerful, have a partner gently touch each area as it is mentioned. Before you begin, go through the instructions below.

Touch the top of the feet; the ankle joint; the top of the shin bones. Cup both hands round the knees in turn; touch the middle of the thigh at the front; then, from behind, place your hands at the top of your partner's leg where it meets the pelvis, the hip joints. Then, standing at your partner's side, place one hand on the back of their sacrum where it meets the pelvis, and one at the front below the belly button; bring the back hand up to the top of the lumbar curve and the front hand to the abdomen, just below the breastbone, then move them up in parallel so that the back hand is touching the back between the shoulder blades, and the front hand is on the breastbone above the breasts. Then place your fingertips at the sides of the neck in the groove behind the ear; place one hand on the top of the head, leave it there for a moment and, as the recording finishes, take the hand away from the head up towards the sky and take a step back from your partner, allowing them to take a walk.

And here are the spoken instructions. An ellipsis (…) denotes the time passing, so that the person standing has time to consider and the person touching has time to change from one site to the next.

'Let's pay attention to the contact force from the earth that is supporting us and taking us up, giving us our full height and stature. As you stand there, supported more on the back of the foot, knees releasing, become aware of the space above you, the space behind you, the space on either side of you, and the space in front of you… Take time to become aware of the ground under your feet… sense the upthrust of the earth itself rising up to the ankle joint… up through the shin bone… up through the knee joints… up through the thigh bones… up through the hip joints… through the inner rim of the pelvis to the front of the sacrum… up through the front of the whole spine, through the lumbar spine… the thoracic spine… the cervical spine, up to where the spine meets the skull… and up to the top of the head… So perhaps it may be possible for you to sense the contact force of the earth all the way up from your feet, up through your ankles, your shin bones, the knees, thigh bones, hip joints, pelvis, the whole of the spine up to the very top of your head… And allow yourself to take a walk, sensing this "up" direction rising up through your very bones as you walk.'

After a moment, return to your partner to share your experience, or return to your logbook to note it down.

Which did you prefer? Paying attention to the gravitational force that connects us downward to the earth? Paying attention to the up direction from the earth? Both are happening at the same time. Gravity, remember, is a force to work *with*, not *against*. Use yourself well with gravity and you will experience yourself with a fluidity, lightness and groundedness.

'If we surrendered
to earth's intelligence

we could rise up rooted, like trees.'

Rainer Maria Rilke[4]

I was often told to find my centre and be grounded. The centre of gravity, the point of balance in a human being, is moving all the time, but generally in relaxed, alert standing the centre is just below your navel, in front of the sacrum. As previously mentioned, 'centre' will be different for different disciplines. The centre we are after here in Alexander Technique is one of easy balance with no effort. As a bit of a space cadet myself I found the 'grounded' instruction not so easy to manage at drama school. In fact, I was a pushover! I was so unaware of the ground, so unaware of my feet, and in a constant, fearful holding pattern. I didn't really know what they meant by 'being grounded', as I had so rarely experienced it. The only time I felt the ground under me was when I had finished bouncing on a trampoline. Then I could really feel the ground come up under my feet. Wow! You can now buy wobble cushions which have the same effect if you stand and balance on them, or walk on the spot on them. Your nervous system has been working so hard with your muscles to keep you balanced that when you step off, the energy still goes on for a while, intensifying the solidity of the ground under your feet. Feel free to get one of these and experiment. The swaying exercise and the previous thinking exercises will help you find your centre and the ground. If you are standing on a train, it's fun sometimes to see if you can balance yourself without having to hold tightly to the bars or straps. The trick is to lower your centre by adopting a wider stance and relaxing into the floor. T'ai chi and qigong are marvellous exponents of this. One of my students who practised aikido once said, 'Ah-ha! So Alexander is like martial arts applied to life!' Here's an exercise I was taught in my t'ai chi classes years ago. I found it very helpful in earthing me – and as an added advantage, it beautifully released my habitual shoulder tension.

Winding Up the Spine

Stand with your feet hip-width apart, knees slightly bent, feet in parallel. Thinking through the suspension system and allowing your thinking to relax you into the ground, keep your gaze and pelvis directed forward, and swing your arms from the front to the back around your torso, to the right and then to the left, giving a passive stretch to the arms and a rotation to the spine. Do not let the pelvis swing round but keep it pointing forward. Do not let the head turn. Do this for about five minutes.

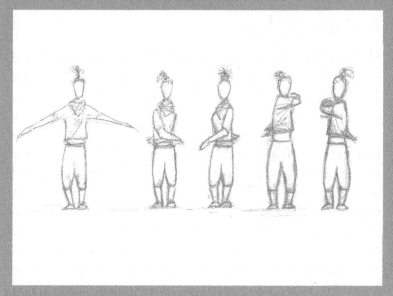

At some point you can alter the swing for a minute to slap the right shoulder blade with your left hand as the back of your right hand smacks the glutes of your left buttock, a diagonal rotation, and vice versa. This is reminding your brain of the cross-over pattern of crawling, improving your coordination at the same time as continuing to energise the spine. Then return to the previous swing. Inhibit the tendency for your legs to inadvertently straighten themselves as you swing. If anything, bend the knees further. Keep your Alexander thinking going; the spatial directions, not trying hard but allowing the movement to happen, keeping the head, neck and back in a dynamic relationship. If you do this in a group or pair, make sure you are facing each other because – when the five minutes is up and you allow your head to lead you up to full standing, so that the legs unfold and straighten – you will be amazed at how your partner or friends appear to rise up strongly and effortlessly. Soloists, use the mirror to observe this in yourself. Go for a walk and I think you might feel the ground underneath you.

Abdominal Muscles

You may have picked up that so far I have not mentioned core muscles. At the time of writing there is a cult which has been going on for some time, certainly since the late 1990s, fuelled by a huge industry and lots of money. It assumes we need to engage the abdominal muscles rigorously all the time. A Feldenkrais friend called core stability 'fascism of the abdomen', as opposed to what we in Alexander land would call 'the cooperation of the head, neck and back'. Here's an interesting fact: the effort needed for our trunk muscles to stabilise us in the simple act of standing is one per cent.[5] You do not need to tighten, contract, pull or push your abdominal muscles to be able to stand in an easy balanced way, so please stop it. You know this is true. If you look at young children, they look cute, have lovely round bellies and are standing perfectly easily without consciously engaging things known as core muscles. You need abdominal muscles for defecating, vomiting, urinating, sneezing, flexing the spine, breathing (as secondary muscles of breathing, I hasten to add) and vocalisation, giving birth, creating abdominal pressure when required, and covering and protecting your internal organs. You do *not* need them to hold yourself up. You may want them to hide the fact you've eaten too much by holding in your tum along with your bum. But, as actors, please don't do this, please, please, pretty please. It doesn't work. (You can hide overeating much more effectively by standing as previously described: by floating the pelvis back and taking yourself out of the banana shape.) As highly educated movers, you will need to do strenuous exercise and be robust, able to flex and extend your trunk, do unusual rotations, etc. Of course, follow your movement teachers' advice and, providing you pause before action, inhibit your reaction and free yourself to the movement, you will be able to do the strengthening and stretching exercises more effectively. But you do not need to be strong to stand, okay? Or to walk. Voice teachers will tell you the same thing: the abdominal muscles need to be flexible, to move, and not to be held or stiff if you want to breathe effectively.

Here's a picture of them, in case you don't know what and where they are, and a good idea to check them out on the internet too.

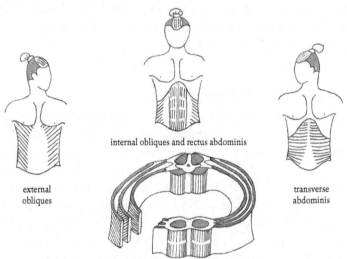

internal obliques and rectus abdominis

external obliques

transverse abdominis

Transverse abdominis is the deepest muscle of them all and holds all the internal organs in place. It can compress the abdomen and create intra-abdominal pressure when needed for certain activities. Next are the internal obliques, followed by the external obliques – both used to rotate and laterally flex the spine. All these muscles are at the sides of the abdomen and are connected to the ribs and pelvis and the connective tissue at the front and back of the abdomen. The rectus abdominis, known as the 'six pack' and connected to pubic bone and ribs, flexes the spine, compresses the abdomen and sometimes emerges as a fashionable 'look', bulging with muscle 'tone'.

It's the shortening and stretching of all these muscles that create the appearance of the mysterious 'waist joint'. If we sit collapsed, over time the muscles shorten themselves, moulding themselves to our use patterns. Stretching them to 'sit up', or 'stand up straight' in the old way is a huge effort for the muscles, which is why we so often collapse down again, pulled into what feels like a more relaxed shape. Not trying to stretch them, but instead engaging with the world so that our head rises as we balance ourselves differently, we free up the muscles gently and begin the process of releasing them back to their optimum length, little by little, much easier to maintain. In this way, the abdominals become a supple web of muscles working together, responding to our needs.

'O, Speak Again, Bright Angel' [6]

Where were we? Oh, yes – now you have learned more about the art of balancing as you stand, allowing yourself to be about to fall, finding the back of your foot, releasing unnecessary tensions in legs and bottom; how to ground yourself and think up at the same time, learned more about your body map and the dear old feet, and to inhibit any extraneous movements as you speak – go back to your original text and try it out in front of the camera or your peers as before. Get some feedback – has something changed? Note it down in your logbook.

Perhaps you have discovered that, by allowing ourselves to let go and come into an ever-changing balance, we achieve great stillness and presence, and our voice takes wing!

Here's what some of my drama students said after their first experience in speaking the Alexander way:

'My voice felt like water pouring out of a jug – a flow to it – effortless.'

'My back is speaking, I can feel the voice coming out of my back!'

'I've never felt anything like that before. I feel a little disorientated – high. It's so unfamiliar.'

Assignments

- Lie down in semi-supine, in either crawling shape as last week or the usual way.

- Practise standing with the two ways of thinking: first, with everything dropping down towards the centre of the earth; and second, with the upthrust from the earth taking you up. Listen to the audio recordings to help guide you.

- For five minutes every day, practise *Winding Up the Spine* to help ground you.

- Walk barefoot in the house and make it foot awareness week. Sway in circles from your ankles. Try wiggling your toes individually. They can all do it eventually, it's just that the neural pathways for that precise wiggling need to be formed. (This might be a long-term experiment...)

- Find the new balance, more on the back of the foot, in your everyday life.

- If it's a windy day, find a nearby tree. Touch it (hugging might get you strange looks) and feel for the movement of the roots creaking as the branches rock in the wind.

- Enjoy freeing the abdominal muscles so you can breathe and balance more easily, and releasing the knees to become even taller.

- And apply all this to speaking your text, inhibiting your usual mannerisms to find your natural vitality and presence.

- Make notes on your progress in your logbook.

- Since the bard has found his way already into this lesson, maybe for next week's experiments learn by heart one of the pieces below from Shakespeare's *King Lear*, or a piece of your own choosing – something similar in its extravagant rage!

'Not only, sir, this your all-licensed fool,
But other of your insolent retinue
Do hourly carp and quarrel, breaking forth
In rank and not-to-be-endured riots, sir.
I had thought by making this well known unto you,
To have found a safe redress, but now grow fearful,
By what yourself too late have spoke and done
That you protect this course and put it on
By your allowance'

Goneril, Act One, Scene Four

'Hear, nature, hear, dear goddess, hear!
Suspend thy purpose if thou didst intend
To make this creature fruitful:
Into her womb convey sterility,
Dry up in her the organs of increase,
And from her derogate body never spring
A babe to honour her, if she must teem,
Create her child of spleen, that it may live
And be a thwart disnatured torment to her'

Lear, Act One, Scene Four

Lesson Seven: The Balancing Act Continues

Experiments in speaking powerfully and emotionally

Equipment

- A peacock feather – or, if you can't find a peacock feather, a long, thin cane
- Space to move, possibly outdoors
- A headrest
- A long mirror
- Your prepared speech
- Phone camera or webcam
- Filming equipment

'At the still point of the turning world. Neither flesh nor
  fleshless;
Neither from nor towards; at the still point, there the
  dance is,
But neither arrest nor movement. And do not call it fixity,
Where past and future are gathered. Neither movement
  from nor towards,
Neither ascent nor decline. Except for the point, the still
  point,
There would be no dance, and there is only the dance.'

T. S. Eliot, 'Burnt Norton'[1]

A Beautiful Balance

Take the long peacock feather and balance it upright on the palm of your hand. Feel free to move around to keep it balancing there. Is it possible to balance it on the tip of your finger? As you look up to the top of your feather, remember to lengthen through your front and use your eyes to lead you, so you are not squashing your neck. Can you change height as you keep it balanced there? Is it possible to dance, keeping your feather upright? Take note of how you are constantly adjusting yourself to keep the feather balanced. You will also notice that at times there is stillness, as though it could stay there poised on your finger forever; a stillness such as a pendulum has when it swings to its limit on one side, in that moment before it changes direction to swing back. So in balance we have movement, and we have stillness.

A peacock feather has only one point to balance on; we generally have two. Our inherent instability is what gives us our energy. A four-legged creature is more stable, but has to use more muscular effort to get around.[2]

How did your assignments go last week? Check out your logbook or check in with your study partner(s). Do you feel more grounded after practising the rotation of the spine? Do you feel more in touch with your feet? Can you sense the up direction through your very bones, even as you allow gravity to root you to the planet? Did you find a tree to touch and sense the roots creaking as the branches rocked in the wind? One lesson I gave on grounding to a boisterous group of musical-theatre students ended with my taking them for a walk to the local park so they could do just that. It was a glorious, windy day, just right for feeling the movement of a tree, and I wanted to take the work out of the classroom. What had that to do with learning about musical theatre? Paul, a very talented student – highly intelligent, alert, very present – questioned this vociferously. I paused and thought for a moment. 'Paul, one day, maybe not for ten years, you will think back to this time, and out of all the lessons you have ever had, not just in Alexander, this is the one that you will remember most and then you will understand.' Ten years later, Paul was back at the theatre school, guesting as a dance tutor. He hailed me excitedly from the other end of the corridor: 'Penny, you were right!'

Have you experimented with leaving your core muscles alone? Have you stopped trying to pull yourself up? Have you allowed yourself to find a new balance more on the back of your foot, with knees unlocked? And that exploration of grounding and centring yourself whilst standing, has that impacted on your text work – have you found more stillness and presence as you speak from the heart?

Speaking with Fury

Record this exercise. Speak aloud one of the pieces from *King Lear* I gave you to prepare. Where is your attention as you speak it? The first time perhaps it was in remembering the words. Speak it again, now you have refreshed your memory, and maintain the thought that the words are coming to you in this moment; you are not going inside to pluck the words from your brain to move to your mouth. Keep your attention out; be spatially aware and, as you speak, let your neck be free, your head releasing forward and up, the back lengthening and widening, the knees unlocked and the feet spreading into the floor, that new Alexander balance. I deliberately chose these speeches because they are not calm, measured pieces but loud, insistent rages that will tempt the old habits out of hiding. Goneril is sick to death of her aged father treating her home like a venue for an all-night party. King Lear is incensed that his daughter could be so ungrateful after he had given her half his kingdom. For a third time, do the speech to your partner, imagined or real, as if they were the character your character is speaking to. Can you inhibit the old patterns? Does your attention narrow to the other, the words, your feelings, or is there still a unified field of attention? Discuss or simply look back at the recording. Which of the three recitations did you prefer?

Let's play with how we can use *The Travelator* to help you stay in your new balanced state.

Running and Hugging

Stand by a wall or tree. Run as hard as you can to a wall or tree opposite you. Turn and run back equally fast, but this time imagine that the wall/tree is coming towards you fast! The travelator we used for walking has speeded up. What happened? It probably felt lighter and more 'up'.

Solo artists – if possible, find someone to play this next part of the exercise with during the week. If you have a partner, label yourselves Rhubarb and Custard. Stand opposite each other, inhibiting and directing. Focus on keeping your attention out and wide, and allow the neck to remain free, letting the head rise, the back to lengthen and widen; with ankle, knee and hip joint unlocked and finding the back of the foot – that's right, the new Alexander balance.

Now here's the story. You and your partner are long-lost friends who have not seen each other for a long, long time. Call their name and wave hello to each other excitedly. Rhubarb, stay where you are; Custard, you're going to run towards Rhubarb and, when you meet, both hug each other. Custard, as you run, imagine Rhubarb coming towards you. Rhubarb, resist the urge to lean forward; wait for Custard to arrive before you give each other the big hug. Ready, steady... Wave! Discuss and swap round.

Perhaps, when you were running, you found that the other person came to you very quickly, easily and the hug just happened? Perhaps when you're standing there waiting for the arrival, it felt unusual. Good – out of habit. Remember, we want to inhabit the unfamiliar, the unknown. When, in real life, would we not anticipate and want to rush forward to greet our friend? If we were unable to move through disability, perhaps. Or if we were of higher status: royalty have someone else dress them – the clothes come to them, the toothpaste is waiting for them on the toothbrush, their servants do the rushing about, whilst they sit sedately on the metaphorical throne.

This time, have both of you do the running, so you meet halfway for a hug, both maintaining the perspective that the other person is coming towards you – this time they really are. Off you go... Amazing how quickly it happens, isn't it? Without effort.

Now let's transform those running rules on the travelator to some text.

Receiving the Words

If you are working on your own, stand opposite your reflection in the mirror, or stand/sit before your own live image on-screen and record it to play it back. Be standing or sitting in your balanced state. I'm going to give you a line of text to say three times. As you speak, have a sense that the text is coming to you from your reflection or the screen image. You are just letting your mouth open to let it out. Ready? Here's the text: I want you to say 'I love you' three times, in your own time. Don't 'do' it, simply allow the words to come. They are coming from the image in front of you on the screen or from the reflection in the mirror. Then play the recording back.

If you are in pairs, stand opposite each other, maybe two arms' length away. Rhubarb, I'm going to give you the line of text to speak three times. Custard, stand there without doing anything. Simply stand in your balanced state, waiting for the text to arrive, waiting to receive it. Rhubarb, I want you too to be standing in the same balanced state and, as you speak, have a sense that the text is coming to you from the other person – you are just opening your mouth to let it out. Here it is: I want you to say 'I love you' three times and in your own time. Don't 'do' it, simply allow the words to come. Swap roles and discuss.

Authentic, powerful and non-doing? The notion of the text coming from the other person, or your reflection, is like the wall or person coming towards you as you run. The impulse to speak comes from them; the words arrive in your brain from the gods and simply spill out of your mouth. Who knows where a thought comes from? Try it again, this time with the words 'I hate you' three times. If in pairs, let Custard do the speaking first, just to change the order. (This is an acting exercise, remember, but if you find it disturbing to be telling someone or yourself that you hate them, feel free to hug them afterwards and make yourself a cup of tea!) Swap and discuss, look back at your recording.

Who said, 'Less is more?'[3] I think this exercise proves it. These are huge emotions, and the words are powerful in themselves if you let them work their magic. Like spells. So often we feel we have to thrust ourselves forward, drop, brace or collapse in order to express ourselves and our emotions authentically to another person. Now you know you don't have to. Words can be spoken clearly and softly but with powerful effect.

Upping the Volume

Well, that's great for film, but suppose you're onstage and need to be on voice?

Cursing

Step away from each other again to create more distance between you, or back off from the mirror or stand away from the screen. Imagine you are at the RSC or the Globe. Let's work with another piece of text: 'May you rot in hell!' (Not a very modern curse, and certainly one with Elizabethan resonances – in Shakespeare's time hell was considered a real place and to damn someone to torture for all eternity is pretty heavy stuff.) Same thing – Rhubarb, stay in your balanced state with that dynamic relationship of the head, neck and back, and bellow this out three times as your partner Custard just stands there, equally balanced, and takes it. And keep imagining that the words and the emotions within the words are coming to you from your partner, reflection or screen image, and you are just opening your mouth and letting them out. Swap and discuss, look back at your recording.

So often, when there's a big speech to be made with added volume, we start poking forward and thinking horizontally. Think instead of going up more, using the up direction from the earth, and staying back. It offers higher status and more control – you can literally see more. And I think you might find that by staying back and up, not interfering with your resonant space or breathing mechanisms, your voice can be easily heard and supported.

One last experiment in speaking powerfully...

Pleading

Come closer together or to the screen or mirror. Speak the text 'Please don't leave me' three times. Abandonment is perhaps our biggest fear: it can be understood and conveyed without doing anything at all. As before, swap and discuss, or play back the recording.

Were they going to leave anyway, despite your plea? It's so easy, when you are pleading and fearful, to drop down and pull your head back. When you do this in front of a mirror, the joy is that you can see the effect of these exercises immediately – the effect of balance, stillness, allowing things to come to you, staying present, not end-gaining. It's a balancing act indeed, to have emotional truth and technique working together. If you are working in a group, I recommend that you sit in a circle after doing these exercises, and have volunteers speak each of the four texts and observe them in performance. We learn so much from others. Soloists, pairs, play the recordings again, make notes in your logbook. See what you see, hear what you hear. Actors used to be the shamans of the tribe. Possessed, we are channelling the spirit of the play, opening our mouths to let out extraordinarily deep and moving experiences. We get out of the way of ourselves.

Infinity and Beyond

Our muscles and connective tissue wind a path up and down our skeleton in such a way that when we leave ourselves alone, we seem to move gently from side to side in a figure-of-eight – the infinity symbol. Try it out.

The Figure-of-Eight

Stand quietly and pay attention to the movement that is your innate instability. Then deliberately sway from your ankles in this figure-of-eight, rather than a circle as in the last lesson. Imagine a plumb line from your coccyx to the earth and make that the marker that is drawing your figure-of-eight on the ground, if that helps. Play with the figure-of-eight one way, and then the other – there will be a dominant rotation and spiral, according to your right- or left-handedness. Allow the movement to become smaller and smaller until you are not doing it at all but just allowing the possibility.

If you are in any doubt about whether you are a whole system, not a cardboard box on two legs, play with the following exercise:

Time to Unwind

Stand in the balanced way and, without moving your feet, look behind you as far as you can, observing what you can see and, with your inner eye, be aware of the degree of rotation happening throughout. Allow yourself to face forward again and you will feel that rush of unwinding. Look behind you the other way, just to balance yourself up.

Balancing is easy. We are finding a balanced way of speaking, of standing, of sitting, of walking.

The Tipping Point

How far can you tip yourself forward or back? Try it out.

Stand in the balanced way and tip forward from your ankles as far as you can, and then tip backwards. I think you will find that you can tip forward from your ankle a long way before a foot moves forward to save you or your knees bend. Tipping backwards you won't go so far. Again, a foot will come back to save you, but it feels inherently unsafe.

We are not designed to fall backward. If we fall forward, our hands will shoot out and our legs organise themselves to save us. When you were walking backwards in Lesson Four, it was easier because you readjusted your whole balance – your head and torso came forward on the hip joint, the pelvis came back in space, just as last week we played with coming out of the banana shape in standing. In fact, that's an easy way to change your balance as you stand. Just imagine you are about to walk backwards, as we did in Lesson Three when exploring Alexander's technique, as you stood and decided whether to speak, not speak or walk backwards. Or imagine you are about to pick something up from the floor. The pelvis, like a pendulum, will swing slightly back in space as the head and torso balance shifts slightly forward.

Semiflexion

When Carnegie Hall in New York was refurbished in 1986, the acoustic changed for the worse. There was some debate as to what had caused this and in 1995 it was discovered that a layer of concrete had been laid under the stage. The concrete was removed and a year later much of the warm, natural acoustic had returned. I like this as a metaphor for our voices. If the stage is the equivalent of our vocal cords, and the resonant chambers of the mouth and pharynx our acoustic chamber, we don't want any concrete below. We need to de-concretise ourselves! No holding tight allowed. Let me continue this notion of balancing rather than having to hold ourselves up by introducing you to what Alexander called the 'position of mechanical advantage' (well, he was Edwardian). You've experimented effectively with semi-supine, half a lying down, so now please welcome semiflexion, a half-standing.

'Halfway down the stairs
is a stair
where I sit.
There isn't any
other stair
quite like
it.
I'm not at the bottom,
I'm not at the top;
so this is the stair
where
I always
stop.'

A. A. Milne, 'Halfway Down'[4]

A great stopping point, halfway down the stairs. The halfway point between sitting and standing is a shape you might also use picking something up or washing your hands. The legs are not fully flexed nor fully extended, but somewhere in the middle. The hip, knee and ankle joints are engaged but not held. The shoulders widening, allowing the arms to gently hang down.

Finding Semiflexion

Stand side-on to a long mirror or the screen. Think of a sport you have taken part in or have watched sufficiently to imitate one of the players – netball, hockey, golf, tennis, basketball. You will find yourself standing with knees bent, torso tipping forward – from the hip joint and not the waist – eyes alert, ready to throw, catch or hit the ball. It is an easy, natural balance for us – tipping forward not backward. Because you are about to run, it's likely that you will find yourself on the front of your foot. Keep the shape but now find the back of the foot. Different? Now think through Alexander's directions – neck free, head forward and up, back lengthening and widening, knees forward and away. Remember the crawling we did to help with your walking, and the crawling shape in semi-supine? This is a standing crawling shape. The spine continues right up to the ears, so no dropping of the neck, and no need to arch the back. Use the mirror or screen to determine if you are in the shape you think you are. Or, in pairs, have one person put their hand on the top of their partner's head and the other on the sacrum as a reference. The distance between the two hands remains the same as the other partner drops over into this halfway place, the arms dangling at the side. Swap over. Experiment always with being aware of your spatial directions, particularly the space above. It will stop you thinking that you're going down, and stooping.

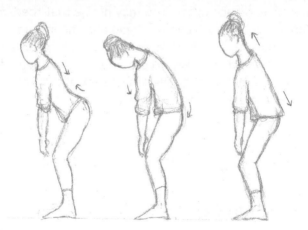

The Golden Chain

As you come into semiflexion, what is leading that movement? Imagine delicately dangling a golden chain between your thumb and forefinger and lowering it onto the palm of your other hand. What happens to the links? The lower ones fold up. So, as the head lowers in space, the legs are like the lower links in the chain; hip, knee and ankle joints coordinating so that they fold up! As you come back up to full standing – raising the golden chain – they unfold. You do not need to push up with your legs; they will unfold to support you as you come back up.

Using the Golden Chain

Experiment with the following two ways and observe the difference. Come into semiflexion by bending the knees and the head following, and come out of semiflexion by pushing up with the legs, head arriving last. Then experiment with the golden chain: head lowering and raising, legs folding and unfolding. Experiment with these two ways again, this time placing the palm of one hand on the back of your head and the back of the other hand on your sacrum. If you are in pairs, place the hands on sacrum and head of your partner as they come into semiflexion in the two different ways, so you can feel the difference in each other. You may notice that there is quite a counterbalance between the head and the sacrum. You have full permission to allow the bottom to lengthen away from the head: it is responding to the weight of the head dropping. Please do not tuck the pelvis in or stick it out. Let your spine and pelvis maintain their integrity.

Speaking from the Halfway House

Humming in Balance

Now let's have you do a simple voice exercise. Stand upright and intone 'Mmmoo, mmmoh, mmmaw, mmmah, mmmay, mmmee.' Now come up and over into semiflexion, and repeat.

If you were standing up 'right' you will have been free, balanced, responsive, on-line and spatially aware, and the difference in the voice between the two positions was perhaps less noticeable. If you were standing 'upright' by fixing and concretising yourself, you will hear and feel quite a resonant shift. I believe that when we are standing in the balanced way, we are already in a 'position of mechanical advantage' – it's just that the angles of the hip, knee and ankle joints are different; the potential for semiflexion is there all the time. There is no difference in your use pattern from standing to sitting to picking something up when we are balancing ourselves easily according to the human form.

Cleaning Teeth

Stand in front of a full-length mirror or screen and pretend for a moment that you are in your bathroom going through the ritual of cleaning your teeth. Mime your regular actions until you have finished the process. If you are in a group or with partners, have one half do the action whilst the other half watches. And swap. What did you observe in yourself or your partner?

Were some of you nearly spitting on the ground as you imagined cleaning your teeth? Our saliva glands certainly get going just thinking about it. (It happens when we imagine eating, too.) When we clean our teeth, even if we have an electric toothbrush, there comes that moment when we need to tip forward so we can spit safely into the basin and not down our front. How did you do that? Did you drop your neck? Did you lock your knees and bend forward at the 'waist joint'? These are all effective ways of carrying out your desire to spit. But how about employing semiflexion? It may feel like a big movement, but this is only because more parts are moving. You are simply balancing yourself throughout the whole of your system to enable the action, taking your space. It's easy to practise in the bathroom because you are on your own and there's no one to make fun of you if you are concerned that your bottom is sticking out more than usual. Often there'll be mirrors in the bathroom to help guide you. And as we generally brush our teeth twice a day, you will be playing with this halfway point at least twice daily. It is easier to do that than if I asked you to think of it every time you sit, stand, pick something up or chew gum throughout the day. This is manageable. Movements can be big, floppy and confident, rather than short, held and self-conscious. Go for it.

Cleaning Teeth to Help the Voice

In front of the mirror, filming yourself or in pairs, mime your teeth-cleaning again, this time using semiflexion. Notice the difference: it doesn't look as silly as it may feel.

Also try changing which hand you hold the toothbrush in from time to time. It will give you a whole different experience of the inside of your mouth. As you play with changing the way you clean your teeth, you will be indirectly doing great work on your voice, de-concretising yourself.

Here's another experiment in helping you speak with knees semiflexed without tilting the torso.

Up Against the Wall

Stand in front of a wall or a door – a smooth, frictionless surface helps. Let your back rest on the wall, with your feet maybe six inches in front, so you can feel your bum and shoulders on the wall. Don't try to push your lower back into the wall; remember we are supposed to have a lumbar curve. Let your head be directed easily up off your spine. Don't try and put the back of your head on the wall: it may reach, but you may be pulling it back. When we lie down we support the head with a block or some books, and this is the same shape as lying down only now you are supported by the wall and the floor. Allow the space behind your knees to increase and you will find yourself sliding down the wall a little way. Keep the heels on the floor. Now allow the space behind your knees to decrease and you will find yourself sliding up the wall. Keep thinking 'up', using the support of the wall and the sense of the planet coming up through your feet. Continue this up direction as your legs are straightening, and then allow the heels to come off the floor as you come up on your toes. Beware – it is not uncommon for the pelvis to suddenly thrust forward as we support ourselves on our toes, so keep it firmly against the wall. We want your hip joints to be working. Allow your heels to gently drop back onto the floor as you slide back down.

Play with this movement of sliding up and down the wall a few times. It helps the brain recalibrate keeping the head, neck and back untroubled as the hip, knee and ankle joints change their angles. Play with speaking the Shakespeare text as you slide up and down. When you finish, do not push yourself off the wall by leading with the pelvis, but lead with your head, tipping the torso forward and sensing the bum still supported by the wall. In this semiflexion, begin the speech again and, as you speak, allow yourself gradually to come up to full standing, and walk until you have finished the speech. This is self-experiment – do not perform the text to someone else at this stage. Give feedback to your partner or make a note in your logbook as to what you experienced.

When we use our leg joints effectively, we stop distorting the torso and become more elegant; we breathe better and come to our full stature. When we brace our legs and are stiffening, we are tightening the hip flexors, the iliacus and psoas muscles, and this pulls on our spine. Time for some more mapping.

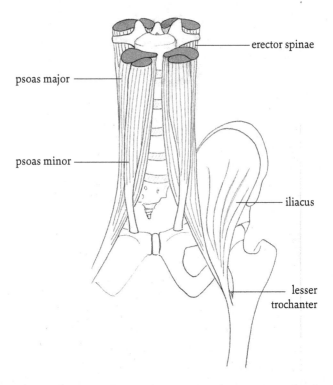

You will see that the psoas major muscle starts at the lesser trochanter, winds a path over the rim of the pelvis and attaches to the side of the lumbar spine. The iliacus starts in the same place but fans out to attach to the top of the pelvis. If these muscles are contracted, they will tilt the pelvis forward and pull on the lumbar spine, overarching the lumbar curve. Psoas minor inserts at the top of the pubic bone and again winds back to join psoas major, attaching to the lumbar vertebra. You will see that these are deep muscles, the psoas muscle nestling against the spine in front of and nearly as thick as erector spinae. It is as though the spine is cradled by these four muscles. They need to be firm and flexible, not shortened and stuck. The only place you can touch the psoas and iliacus is in the groin area: after that they dive behind your intestines. But you can feel the effect of them in the lower back.

Psoas to Free Your Hip Joints

As you stand, place one hand on your lower back at the side of the lumbar spine and one in the groin area (same side). Deliberately tighten your knees back and tense the legs and you may feel the effect that has on your lumbar spine. You may also note that your breathing is affected. Where the muscle fibres of the psoas stop, the fibres of the diaphragm begin. They are functionally connected. Now release the legs, allowing the knee to come forward a little and come to balanced standing. You may feel the lower back release into your hands, the pelvic tilt reorganise and the breath let go. Play with this in pairs if you can. Those of you with a healthy, flexible psoas may notice less difference.

How to remember the name of this muscle? It is there 'so-as' to free the hip joint. It is a bridge between the legs and the lumbar spine. What will free the psoas if it is habitually contracted? All the things we are working with now – finding a freely movable, balanced standing, lying in semi-supine, practising semiflexion. There are also some special stretches you can do for psoas.[5] The most Alexandrian is to kneel on one knee, tuck the pelvis under so the spine is not arched, and gently lean in to the leg in front. You will feel it in your groin and thigh. Try it for maybe a minute each side – that will be enough to give you an idea. It is a stretch I learned from Malcom Balk, an Alexander running coach.[6] Alexander Technique can help make all exercises more effective by not trying hard, inhibiting your immediate reaction to the movement, and directing yourself consciously.

Head to the Wall

Come onto your hands and knees and reprise the crawling we did in the lesson on walking, starting with rocking forward and back before setting off. Crawl towards a wall. Place a foam headrest or a paperback book between the top of your head and the wall, directing the top of your head into the wall so the headrest stays put. Your hands are pointing forward, arms not braced, supporting under the shoulder, but with most of the weight going down through the thighs, with knees under the hip joints. Intone: 'Mmmoo, mmmoh, mmmaw, mmmah, mmmay, mmmee.' Gently roll your head back so that the contact with the wall is now your forehead. You will feel that your neck is shortening and your back more likely to be arched. Intone again: 'Mmmoo, mmmoh, mmmaw, mmmah, mmmay, mmmee.' Feel and hear a difference? Gently roll the head back so that the top of it is in contact with the wall again. Take one hand off the floor for a moment and you will feel the head and the other three limbs compensate, but maintain the direction through the top of the head so that the headrest stays in place. Replace the hand and repeat with the other limbs. Does it make a difference if you lift the knee up and forward slightly, or lengthen it back? Attain an even balance as before and speak your Shakespeare text. Allow the weight of your bum to drop you back on the heels, so that you are facing the wall. You are likely to feel your head rising up from your spine as the pressure on the head has been released. Use the wall to crawl upwards towards standing. Say the speech *sotto voce* in semiflexion, then turn outwards, gently coming to full standing whilst keeping the quality of semiflexion. Perform the piece to the mirror or camera, or perform to your original partner. Give feedback or look at the recording, discuss, make notes in your logbook.

Has all that work we've done on not end-gaining – allowing the words to spill out, finding a healthy balance in your standing – impacted on your vocal resonance, interpretation and delivery of the lines? These are experiments, and some may work better for you than others. Whatever you have discovered is entirely valid.

More Experiments with the Halfway Point

Halfway Up or Halfway Down?

Come into semiflexion as best you can (which does not mean try hard to get it right but simply to have a go at this new coordination). As you balance there, think about coming back up to full standing, then decide instead that you are going to pick something up from the floor. Can you feel how your intention changes the effort? The thought of coming up lightens it for me.

To begin with, I found semiflexion very awkward and weird – surely my bottom was sticking out? But once I realised that it wasn't a position but simply a chosen balance – a moment in time before I moved, a pendulum swing – I found it much easier. As Alexander said, 'There is no such thing as a right position, but there is such a thing as a right direction.'[7] And it's great for playing with your inhibition skills.

Simply Changing Shape

As you go to pick up an object from the floor, pause and instead think of coming up to full standing before you pick up the object. Remember you are not going down. Since you exist all the way to your feet and the feet are not sinking down through the floor, you are just changing shape. As you rise up with the object, take in the space around, noticing how the spatial parameters are changing as you move through space. How was that?

Notice how a child goes to pick something up from the floor and you will see that the legs are automatically released to allow a full squat. Like cleaning the teeth, it may seem like an enormous movement for a relatively small action or a small object. That's fine – let it be big and released, take your space. Inhibit tightening the arms as you come up, and allow the object to rise up with you. Yes, it does work, even with quite big or heavy things. If you are doing a get-in or get-out this week, that's perfect to play with semiflexion!

Assignments

- Lie in semi-supine. Play with speaking some text as you lie there. Does the head move from side to side or is it pulled back into the headrest? Or can it just rest there as you speak? Lie still again and stay with your spatial awareness, non-doing practice. At the end, have another go: is it different? If you can sense tightening as a prep for speaking, is it possible to inhibit? Give yourself permission not to speak, to think perhaps of raising an arm instead and then speak... The floor and the headrest will give you instant feedback.

- Practise semiflexion as you clean your teeth.

- Practise inhibition as you use semiflexion to pick things up.

- Experiment with leaning your back into the wall and slide slowly up and down.

- Crawl to a wall and use the contact between the head and the wall to help you find that connection between the head, neck and back. Incorporate both these in your vocal warm-ups and text work.

- Revise again the world coming towards you – as in *The Travelator* – as you walk or as you run.

- Look up more pictures on psoas and iliacus on the internet and experiment with the exercises if you feel your own hip flexors need attention.

- Allow yourself to feel the figure-of-eight instability as you stand. Allow yourself to balance in the still point, rather than holding a standing position.

- And keep your spatial awareness going!

'Speak the speech, I pray you, as I pronounced it to you, trippingly on the tongue: but if you mouth it, as many of your players do, I had as lief the town-crier had spoke my lines. Nor do not saw the air too much with your hand, thus, but use all gently; for in the very torrent, tempest, and, as I may say, the whirlwind of passion, you must acquire and beget a temperance that may give it smoothness.'

Hamlet, Act Three, Scene Two[8]

Lesson Eight: Let the Breath Move You

Belief systems of breathing, mapping the breathing mechanisms, and experiments to free it all up

Equipment

- A device with internet access
- Print-outs or photocopies of outline of the body from page 192
- A pen
- A mat
- A headrest

'I see at last that if I don't breathe, I breathe...'

F. M. Alexander[1]

How's your semiflexion? Are your teeth cleaner this week? Haha! Is it feeling a little more natural to counterbalance head and bum? Remember, young children use it all the time. They never pick things up by bending over from the waist. How were the experiments in speaking whilst lying in semi-supine? If you've been practising some text work, how useful were the experiments in allowing the words to come to you? Share with your study partner or reflect in your logbook. You are almost certainly becoming more and more familiar with allowing yourself to balance, rather than holding yourself up.

Even if you are balancing on two legs by fixing, tightening and drawing yourself up, trying to be as still as possible, you cannot help but be moving: if you were not moving you would faint, or be dead. We can do without food for few weeks, water for a few days, but without oxygen we can only manage minutes. We are all moving all the time, asleep or wake – we are moved by the air entering and exiting our lungs, like swing doors responding to the wind, like the opening and closing of a paper bag, the air flows in and the air flows out, irregularly as the waves on the shore. Best of all, most of the time it happens without us having to do a thing! It is organised by the autonomic nervous system: like the heartbeat, it just happens all by itself, according to the air pressure and the register of carbon dioxide and oxygen levels in the blood. If we need more oxygen to walk up a hill or run, the rate of air inhalation and exhalation changes by itself. We don't have to do it consciously. It responds to the environment and to our activity. Air molecules rush into the alveoli in the lungs, where the gas exchange takes place, and by the elastic recoil of the lungs and surface tension, the air is expired. In relaxed breathing, it is a passive movement. Nature abhors a vacuum, so as one is created by the retreat of the air, the air will easily rush back in to fill the lungs.

'We live at the bottom of an ocean of air under considerable pressure, which is all too happy to force itself into our lungs, pushing them out against the chest wall.' David Gorman[2]

The air molecules are the bottom layer of the planet's atmosphere and they travel around – the air molecules you are breathing in as you read this may have been in the lungs of a Maori fisherman last week. We share the air of our planet with all living things, including the trees and the vegetation of the earth, balancing the composition of the gases to allow us to coexist. It comes in through the nose or mouth – faster through the mouth – and out through the same organs. The nose warms the air as it enters, and takes out some of the impurities. If we have a cold and our nose is blocked, our mouth takes over automatically. As athletes of the voice, actors are learning to control this vital movement just like swimmers, singers and wind-instrument players. And it is our out-breath that moves us. It is air travelling through our vocal cords that gives us sound. And mostly (but not always), we make sound from the air travelling out of the lungs. Have a go at doing it the other way, making a sound as you breathe in – say the word 'yuh' on the in-breath. Nordic and Icelandic readers, you will find this very familiar – it is the way of assenting, saying yes, on the in-breath. Experiment with speaking a whole sentence on the in-breath. Not quite so resonant, eh? Best stick to the out-breath for Shakespeare.

There She Blows

Blow all the air out of your lungs. (I bet most of you take an in-breath for some weird reason before you start expelling the air!) As you get to the end of the exhale, stop the airflow for a moment and then let it rush back in. Put one hand on your breastbone, the back of the hand on the back of the ribs at the top of the lumbar spine and repeat, so you can feel this movement with your hands. Pairs, you can feel this on your partner: take it in turns to place hands on each other in the same way, only now you will be able to use the palm of your hand instead of the back. Ask them to breathe out and then let the air rush back in. Do this again, but this time place the hands at the side of their ribs.

If you want to hold your breath for any reason, it's much easier to do it on the out-breath, as the air will come in much faster than if you hold it on the in-breath. You have to spend time breathing out to allow the space for the new air to come in. Play with comparing the two. A quick in-breath is a gasp made through the mouth, associated with the fear response. In contrast, a long out-breath is a letting go, an expiration, a relaxation, a pleasurable sigh... If you are intending to say a long sentence, your out-breath will adapt and become longer. Many voice exercises use this natural organisation – such as counting to five, then ten, then fifteen, twenty, twenty-five... as you increase the out-breath little by little. This practice allows you to maintain a consistent airflow to the end of the sentence. It exercises the muscles of the breathing apparatus, so you use them fully and easily. Supporting the breath does not mean holding or tightening any muscles, but allowing them to engage in such a way that the outward airflow is controlled over a longer time frame, and it's for you to choose when to let the air come back in. You could say that if the intention is clear, the thought organises the breath and 'propels the sound'.[3] Like all athletes, if you are not practised in sustaining the out-breath, you are less able to realise your thought. As you practise, you will increase your lung capacity so it all becomes much easier.

Where the Air Actually Goes

Let us check your map of the breathing apparatus. There is so much imagery used in exploring the art of breathing, from yoga to singing, our individual maps can be wildly inaccurate. And as you know by now, your belief systems can affect how well you function.

Where are the Lungs, Trachea and Diaphragm?

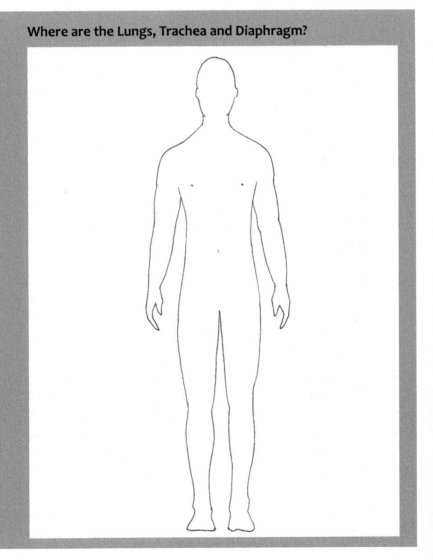

If working in a group, it's best to have prepped this by having copies of the drawing for everyone. Either download and print from www.nickhernbooks.co.uk/alexander-technique, or photocopy the previous page. Draw in where you think the lungs, the windpipe and the diaphragm are. Study partners, compare your drawings. Now look at the back of the book in Appendix B and compare your drawing with the one there. Ah-ha! Please also check out 'lung position in ribcage' online and look at the images there.

You will find that the lungs are pear-shaped, they start *above* the collarbone and there is more lung tissue at the back of you than in the front. There is more lung tissue on the right side than the left because the left needs to make room for the heart, which sits on top of the diaphragm on the left. The bottom of the lungs at the front is level with your sixth rib, where the bra strap is, much higher up than folks often realise. The diaphragm is not a flat disc at the front of the abdomen, it is a dividing muscle which separates the airtight thoracic cavity from the abdomen. It's a half-mushroom or umbrella shape, domed, the stalk attached to the first two or three vertebrae of the lumbar spine, with the edges of the diaphragm fanning out to attach to the tip of the breastbone and the bottom of the ribs, right round to the back. Originally, in our evolution from fish, the diaphragm would have been the long muscle at the front of the spine: as the gills developed into lungs, the lungs budded down and peeled the front muscle off the spine. This then spread out to attach to the ribs, folding over the vital organs – liver, spleen, stomach – with the end of that front muscle still latched onto the lumbar spine. The vital organs are protected by the diaphragm and also get a nice massage as they are displaced by its action. If the ribs are restricted, the wall of the abdomen will need to push out in front much more. The diaphragm has to find 'give' somewhere and will push further down on the vital organs if the ribs aren't moving. Find the bottom of your breastbone. The dome of the diaphragm never goes below that point. The edges of the diaphragm never invert the shape; they are gently directing the ribs outwards to increase the volume of the thorax.

Take out your devices now and watch this animation of the diaphragm on YouTube.[4] (youtu. be/hp-gCvW8PRY)

I used to get my knickers in a twist about what the diaphragm and ribs were doing until my Alexander trainer came in one morning with a paper bag and demonstrated the action of the thoracic cavity: open the bag and the air flows in, close the bag the air flows out – the diaphragm is the bottom, the ribs the sides, and the bag is opening and closing continuously. The air isn't being sucked in or pushed out, it just flows easily. Suddenly it all made sense! Of course the thoracic cavity is not empty like a bag, it is filled with lungs and the heart. The incoming air, filled with oxygen that brings life to us, travels from the world via the nose or mouth, down the trachea, the bronchii and into the lungs. The lungs are like a root network; spongy, elastic, fibrous tissue with tubes and air sacs. They have a huge surface area – laid out they would fill half a tennis court! The air sacs, or alveoli, interface with blood capillaries to receive oxygen from the outside world and expel carbon dioxide. The air filled with carbon dioxide travels from this root system, along the bronchii to the trachea or windpipe, and up into the world via your nose or mouth. This is the air you are using to make sounds with. The trachea is made up of rings of cartilage. The larynx is simply a specialised part of the trachea, at the top, and the vocal folds (or cords as they are often called) are two bands of ligament that lie horizontally across the trachea. These are tiny: only 12.5mm to 25mm long, depending on size and gender.

———

————

actual length of vocal folds

The folds open and close to prevent food getting down the air passage, and conveniently help to make sound by restricting the airflow. Just to be clear: the vocal folds sit horizontally in the trachea or windpipe.

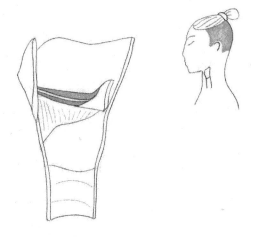

Check out vocal folds on an internet search to get more illustrations and more information on how they work. If you place your fingertips on either side of the larynx you will find you can move it from side to side a little. Keep your fingers there and turn your head. You will find that the larynx is still – a wonderful suspension system of muscles is ensuring it is not distorted during movement.

Ribs

The ribs are pairs of thin, curved bones, connected with freely movable joints to the twelve thoracic vertebrae of the spine. Between them are the internal and external intercostal muscles. Each rib moves differently from the one above and the one below it. The ones nearer the top allow for a movement that raises the front; those nearer the bottom to swing up and out to the side. (Fortunately, they all move in formation at the same time!) Apart from the 'floating' ribs at the bottom, the ribs are connected to the breastbone at the front by cartilage.

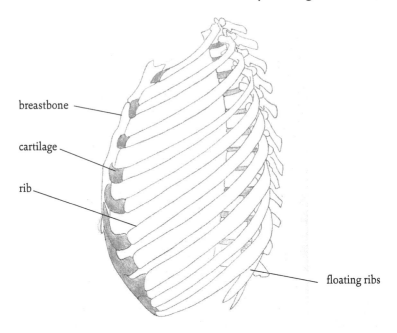

The breastbone is shaped like a necktie with three segments: the knot, the body of the tie and the upside-down triangle at the end, called the xyphoid process. That means that the breastbone also has 'give' in it and can move along with the ribs. The two pairs of floating ribs at the back are shorter, and connect only to the spine and the diaphragm. They are the ones that easily get pushed forward and narrowed as we arch our lumbar spine. They are released when we stand well or use semiflexion.

Get your devices out now and check out this short extract from the animation *The Art of Breathing* by Alexander teacher Jessica Wolf. It shows beautifully the movement of the ribs, the breastbone, the diaphragm, the placement of the vital organs and the muscles involved in breathing.[5] Watch it several times. (youtu.be/apFui6-ffnM)

Restricting the Ribs

Lie on a mat on the floor in semi-supine and with headrests, and notice how your abdomen is moving as you breathe. The movement of your ribs is compromised because you are lying on the back of them. You will notice much more movement at the front of the ribs and the abdomen. Turn over and lie on your right side. Perhaps you can feel how the left side of your ribs, front and back, is now free to move, whilst the right side is restricted? Try it out on the other side, too. Now roll over onto both knees, bum dropped onto your ankles, supporting your forehead by your two fists. In this foetal position, the front of your ribs are more restricted and you are likely to sense much more movement in the back of the ribs, as the whole back is lengthening. Isn't it brilliant how, despite parts of our thoracic cavity being restricted, the rest compensates?

Voice teachers often emphasise the movement of the lower ribs along with the diaphragm, particularly at the back, to ensure a fuller breath, but they are not suggesting that the breastbone and upper ribs be still: everything is moving to allow the air to enter and exit. The shoulder blades, sitting behind the ribs on your back, will also move, as you saw on that last film. The main breathing muscles are the diaphragm and the intercostal muscles. Secondary to that are arm, neck and abdominal muscles. When you blew all your air out, you will have noticed the exertion of the abdominal muscles. The fibres of the transverse abdominis interdigitate with the diaphragm. Given that we need the abdominal muscles to be free to respond to the inspiration and expiration, it's ironic that at the same time there is this culture of strengthening them to hold you upright. Hmmm.

I repeat: abdominal muscles are secondary muscles of breathing, not primary. I also want to refer back to the psoas muscle I introduced in the last chapter on page 180, the thick hip flexor that acts as a bridge between the leg and the spine.

You felt the tightening in the lower back when you braced the legs, the release in that area when you stopped bracing, and how that tightening effected the breath. Where the muscle fibres of the psoas stop, the fibres of the diaphragm begin.

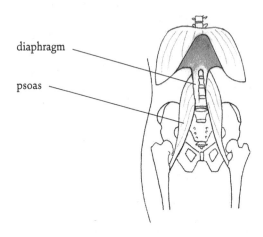

diaphragm

psoas

Best not to hold abdominals or legs if we want to breathe easily. A Chinese saying, often quoted by t'ai chi masters, maintains that 'The ordinary man breathes through the throat, the wise man breathes through the soles of his feet.' I would like to say, 'The wise woman is breathed through her whole self.' Because there is so much movement throughout our system as we breathe, people use a lot of imagery to convey what is happening. Perhaps we are instructed to send the breath into the abdomen or the pelvic floor; or imagine the breath dropping down like water into a huge lake, the water rising up a well, and so on. Whatever floats your boat. If they work for you, feel free to use these images and metaphors. But the truth is that the gas exchange happens where your lungs are, and they are up top. You cannot get the air to drop into your abdomen; it simply is not possible. There are no air sacs in the abdomen, there is only the digestive system – and we know what happens when we get air in that! Another student of mine was not moving his upper chest. He was stressed and breathing quite shallowly. I asked where he thought his lungs were. He pointed to somewhere low down in his abdomen. I placed my hands on either side of his breastbone and asked what he thought was there. He looked perplexed and confessed he didn't know. He was flabbergasted when I told him, and suddenly his whole thoracic cavity started moving again. Perhaps having a more accurate sense of your breathing apparatus might help you to breathe more easily, too. Let's find out.

Mindfulness of Breathing

This is a meditation practice I learned at the London Buddhist Centre many years ago. It's an excellent practice in inhibition, too. When we direct our attention to our breathing it is difficult not to interfere with it, particularly if, as actors, we have spent time trying to control it. Breathing is organised by our autonomic system, but the somatic nervous system gets involved as we direct the airflow. Here is a five-minute meditation exercise in witnessing without interfering. The conscious mind is witnessing the autonomic system without the somatic nervous system reacting. Not so easy!

Mindfulness of Breathing

Using your Alexander thinking so you are directing yourself, sit on a chair, supported by the sitting bones, feet easily supported by the ground in front of you, legs with some space between them. Let your hands rest comfortably on the top of your thighs – I suggest palm up, as this allows greater width of the chest and shoulders, whilst maintaining an up direction through the bones of the arm. Please use the back of the chair if you need support, and use a book or cushion at the back of your thoracic spine if the back of the chair tips you back too much. Let your eyeline drop towards the floor, or close your eyes. Count ten in-breaths. If you lose count, start again from number one. When you have reached your tenth in-breath, count ten out-breaths. If you lose count start again from number one. When you reach your tenth out-breath, count ten whole breaths. If you lose count go back to number one. When you reach your tenth whole breath, stop counting and bring your awareness to the movement of the breath and the breathing apparatus. After about a minute, shift your attention to the gateway of the breath – where you can feel the entrance and exit of the breath. Mouth or nose, it does not matter which, or maybe the air enters through one and exits through the other. Whichever you are using, it is a portal between the outside world and the inside world. We are allowing the outside world to enter us and to leave us. You may even notice the nasal cycle, that one nostril is taking in more air than the other. This is a cycle that changes every two and a half hours on average. Observe the portal for about a minute. Then allow your eyes to open or extend your vision away from the floor, taking in the rest of the world. Please discuss or note your experience. I suggest you practise this for at least five minutes every day.

You Need Never Take a Breath Again

Alexander was known as 'The Breathing Man', the guy you went to if you wanted to improve this aspect of your life, yet he gave few exercises in breathing. He reckoned it was of primary importance to have a dynamic head–neck–back relationship, that gave freedom of movement to the whole self; to be well balanced, to be well grounded and 'up'. If the whole system is working well, then the breath will be coming and going naturally and easily. As my teacher David Gorman writes:

'It is the freedom of the parts that allows free breathing, and free breathing is the opening of the torso into volume. Free breathing is also openness to what's around you. It is you letting the outside into you and allowing what's in you to get out. It is animation and activity, expression and response.'[6]

LESSON EIGHT: LET THE BREATH MOVE YOU

When Alexander was sure all the freeing-up had been addressed, he would then apply the work to breathing and vocal habits where necessary.

> 'When I ask you to draw your tongue away and say "t", I mean you not to say "t". I mean you definitely to prevent, to give orders and not to say "t". I ask you to say "t" because I don't want you to say "t", because I want to give you the opportunity of refusing to say "t".'
> F. M. Alexander[7]

Lovely inhibition again. He also used whispered vowel sounds. Whispering would help disentangle the habitual misuse of the vocal mechanisms by still engaging the vocal cords but taking away the need to be heard, to 'do' speaking. It would allow the person to focus on the step-by-step process, rather than on the goal of 'making a sound'. He experimented with all the vowel sounds but favoured the whispered 'ah', as it allowed a wider, fuller release of the resonant space, lowering the tongue and sending the soft palate up. (There are reasons why a doctor asks you to say 'ah' as she looks down your throat!) The whispered 'ah' is like an upward sigh. Often sighs can take us into a collapse, starting with a breath in to hoik us up, and a collapse down as we let go the breath. Alexander's whispered 'ah' maintains the dynamic relationship of the head, neck and back. And it proves again that, when we let go the air, it will come back in quite easily.

Alexander's Whispered 'Ah'

Stand in your now familiar more balanced way, and think of something funny. 'Last night I dreamed I was eating a giant marshmallow. When I woke in the morning my pillow was gone!' (Thanks, Tommy Cooper!) Okay, something else. It could be thinking of something naughty, or a joyful thing – anything

201

that brings a natural smile to the face. Not a big laugh, that's too much, but a gentle, genuine smile. As the smile spreads over your face, open your jaw, place the tip of your tongue behind the bottom teeth and allow the air to exit on a whispered 'ah'. Then close your jaw and let the air back in through your nose. Do not do more than three of those at one time, or you may hyperventilate. Keep the smile going throughout. Do not breathe in to start the exercise, just let out whatever air is there as you open the jaw. It doesn't have to be the longest out-breath you have ever known. Remember, the smile has to be genuine. If it's genuine, the false folds also open and won't interfere with the passage of air. Thinking of something funny also disrupts the mental attitude of 'This is hard work, I have to concentrate and try hard!', and we release the muscles of the face and jaw. As we discovered in Lesson Three, the jaw is at the front of the neck and needs to open easily to let the breath out.

Experiment with whispering on the other vowels. Remember the recipe: directing up, thinking of something funny, smiling, tip of tongue behind bottom teeth, opening the jaw, letting the air out on the whisper, closing the jaw and allowing the air in through the nose. Was Alexander right – is 'ah' the best one? I recommend a whispered 'oo' if your top lip doesn't like to move very much – the stiff-upper-lips, cockney sparrers, ventriloquists or smilers among you. It's a very curious sensation to smile and 'oo' at the same time! Disrupts the habit nicely.

Here's a singing experiment with the whispered 'ah' – as you know, singing has even more need for the sustaining of the out-breath.

The Whispered 'Ah' for Singing

Think of a line from a song with a high note that you might sometimes have difficulty with. If singing is not your thing that's okay, try it anyway for experiment's sake – you don't have to be in tune, just pick a note, any note. Mime it. Or prepare to sing it but don't let the sound come out. (If you are working in a group or pair, do this all at the same time.) What was happening? Perhaps you noticed some unnecessary tension due to the anxiety of singing a little out of your range. I am now giving you the opportunity of refusing to sing this note! Instead, think of something funny, whisper an 'ah' as instructed above and, after the air has whooshed back in through your nose, sing the note. What do you think? It certainly puts an end to the old habit of sucking in air to prepare for a vocal challenge. Discuss.

More on the Jaw

The whispered 'ah' is a great one for releasing the jaw. Did you find yourself yawning afterwards? Yawning is always good for stretching those jaw muscles. When someone yawns it allows others to yawn. Yawning in Alexander lessons is never offensive – it often happens after a whispered 'ah' and it is getting everything nice and open. Let's remind ourselves of that hinge and slide action of the jaw we covered in Lesson Three. Get your devices out and look at this YouTube video of the joint and movement of the jaw.[8] (youtu. be/p-cW4a8i5_E)

Allowing Your Head to be Still

Place your hands on the joint just in front of the ear, and open and close the jaw slowly a few times, feeling that forward and down motion. Now deliberately hold your jaw in place and move the head up from it saying, 'Can I speak like that?' Answer: yes, but what a lot of effort! There are some among you (you know who you are!) who like to move the head to speak. Replace your hands on the side of your head and say the same thing, keeping the head still and letting the jaw open. So much easier.

The following exercises can help inhibit the extraneous head movement by working the jaw muscles and stretching the tongue.

Using Your Tongue to Release the Jaw

This first one is also useful if you have a habitual asymmetrical movement of the jaw, pulling to one side. Place the tip of the tongue at the back of the teeth as in the whispered 'ah', but this time push the blade or centre of the tongue forward so it sticks out between your teeth, and then let it retreat again. In this way the movement is taken by the tongue leading and the jaw following as it opens and closes. Do ten of those at a time – no rush, in your own time.

Here's a more light-hearted way to release restrictive muscles of the jaw. Speak the days of the week as usual. Then speak them again with the tongue stuck out between the teeth. As you speak, be careful you don't start nodding your head or retracting the tongue. Keep it out there! It will sound daft, but boy does it liberate the jaw and lips as they work hard to substitute for the articulation of the tongue. Now bring the tongue back in and speak the days of the week again. Hear the difference? Not only in the articulation but in the resonance. We need a free jaw to let the air out, and it changes the shape of the mouth, one of the main resonating chambers.

Breathing to Maintain Your Length

Another misconception is that when we breathe out we get shorter and when we breathe in we get taller. Just for a moment try that out: breathe in and pull the chest and shoulders up, and breathe out and collapse. Rather like the sighing I wrote about earlier. When you blow all the air out you will feel your chest cavity getting smaller, and then when the air rushes back in, there's a huge expansion. If we literally had to get taller and shorter, we would be bobbing up and down all the time. Take a look at some other people in the room or out of the window. Can you see if they are bobbing up and down? No. Even if someone is slumped on a chair, their downward direction tends to be unmoving. The spine is flexible and moves as we breathe, the same as the rest of our body. It is more useful to think of your whole self getting longer as you breathe out. Look at Jessica Wolf's animation of breathing again. Your ribs are swinging inwards and down so the air has got to be flowing up and out. The air is rising, the diaphragm is rising, the heart is rising... In martial arts, the forceful kick or arm-swing is done on the out-breath, often with a voice to it: 'O!'

Move on the Breath

Let's go back to our previous experiments with semiflexion and picking things up. Play first with breathing in as you pick something up, secondly holding the breath as you do it and then thirdly breathing out as you do it. Which is easier? Perhaps the best way is not to think about it but trust that it will simply organise itself as you move? Experiment with this again in pairs or using the mirror. Place your hands again at your own or your partner's head and sacrum, and this time deliberately think of maintaining the length of the torso as you pick something up on the out-breath. Discuss your findings or note it down in your logbook.

In the last lesson, when you were speaking emotionally at some volume, perhaps you noticed that habitual tendency to push the head and neck forward, and shorten your stature. If instead your brain associates the out-breath with lengthening the stature, it may help to sabotage the old reaction and keep the head going up rather than forward as you speak. Even experiments in picking things up can help your voice!

Think on the Breath

Lie down in semi-supine again for a moment. As the air enters, imagine your awareness coming in at your feet, and then exiting the feet as you breathe out. On the next in-breath, allow the awareness to come into your feet and legs, and out again as the air flows out. As you breathe in, allow your awareness to spread up through your feet, your legs and your torso, and out again as you breathe out. Next time, as you allow the air to enter, allow the awareness to spread up through the feet, the legs, the torso and the arms, and all the way out as you breathe out again. Next time allow your awareness to spread up through your feet, your legs, your torso, your arms and your neck and head – and out again. Repeat this last full spread of consciousness in time with your breath for a little while. So with every in-breath you are gathering your awareness, receiving your conscious self; and as you breathe out, you're letting it all go.

Letting it go is really important. We so often think 'Now I have that lovely, open, free, effortless feeling, how do I keep it?' The answer is to let it go, so it can come back again. It will stop you trying to hold on to it and thereby losing it anyway.

> 'The experience you want is in the process of getting it. If you have something, give it up. Getting it, not having it, is what you want.' F. M. Alexander[9]

> 'He who binds to himself a joy
> Does the winged life destroy
> But he who kisses the joy as it flies
> Lives in eternity's sunrise.'
>
> William Blake[10]

As usual, we've covered a lot this lesson. A trip around your beliefs on the breath, the breathing apparatus and the jaw; some experiments in breathing for vocal ease, to expand your awareness, and to make it easier to pick things up. Have fun experimenting with all of that this week, and in letting it go!

Assignments

- Semi-supine, synchronise your awareness with your breathing.

- Look at the anatomy pics of the breathing apparatus from time to time. Maybe print them out and stick them on your wall. Check out the internet for pictures and videos of the breathing mechanisms.

- Practise *Mindfulness of Breathing* for as long as you like, but at least five minutes every day. Meditation can go on for hours.

- Pause and, as you use semiflexion to clean your teeth, allow the air to flow out.

- When you want to pick something up, pause and allow the movement to happen consciously on the out-breath.

- Practise *Alexander's Whispered 'Ah'* three times, three times a day. Practise it if someone slights you or annoys you – inhibit your reaction. Instead of gritting your teeth and counting to ten, direct yourself up, think of something funny, etc. (Better make the smile on your face a small, barely noticeable one so as not to offend the other person!)

- Jot down your discoveries in your logbook.

Lesson Nine: Effortless Movement

Floating upstairs and downstairs, in and out of chairs, and a voyage around your arms

Equipment

- A cardboard box or washing-up bowl that you can step into (a shoebox is too small)
- Access to a nearby staircase
- A device with internet access
- A tape measure
- A chair
- A table
- A mirror
- A wall
- Your recording device

'The knots in our hearts keep us from
Crying and dancing when we long to –
They tie us to the posts of the fences
That separate us from each other
The knots in our muscles keep our teeth clenched
Our jaws locked, our legs crossed, our shoulders
Stooped, our backs bent, our chests from
Inhaling and exhaling the full sweetness
Of life's breath.
O, God, untie all those knots!'

Sheila Peltz Weinberg[1]

A Warm-up Sing-song

As a warm-up, sing the song 'Summertime' out of tune.[2]
Remember to pause to redirect yourself, giving yourself the
opportunity of not doing this; perhaps walking backwards
instead, perhaps doing a whispered 'ah' first and then, as the
air comes back in, off you go. If you don't know 'Summertime',
choose another well-known ditty that has passion and
meaning behind it. Irreverently choosing not to sing in tune
takes the pressure off trying to get it right, whilst practising
your Alexander inhibition and direction. After a while, just
the thought of a whispered 'ah' will make you smile, as you
associate it with being light-hearted and fun!

How were this week's joyous experiments in allowing yourself
to be breathed? Have you explored the internet for more
images and information? Have you stuck up some pictures of
the breathing apparatus around your home to remind you?
The back of the loo door is often a useful place. You could also
change the wallpaper on your devices to something relevant
to breathing. Please discuss your experiments, or read through
your logbook and reflect on your learning. I realise that there is
a lot of new input each week and it may not be possible to carry

out all the experiments, but better to have too many than too few. Remember, it's good for the brain to be given a lot to think about, as the little it manages will be more than any one thing that you focus on. You can learn easily without even being aware of the learning, I promise.

Here's a fun experiment in balance and movement that will really help you and will never be forgotten. 'I'm still thinking of stepping into cardboard boxes, Penny!' say my drama students on Facebook, years after they have left drama school. It was inspired by the college stairs – we were on the second and third floor of the building – and I taught it fairly early on as a means of applying inhibition easily and effectively to the movement of walking up stairs, so that they could arrive without being out of puff.

Walking Upstairs

First, come onto all-fours, adjusting your balance as we have done before and, with your head leading, rock forward and back a couple of times to ensure you are freeing the hip joint and extending your head up and away from the shoulders, so that your neck is not dropping. Please take your time and bring awareness to what you are doing and how you are doing it. Then, on your next rock back, start crawling backwards. Remember not to lift your leg but let the shin slide along the floor. Then pause and bring yourself to standing – not with a roll-up! Sit back on the heels, feet flat so you are vertical, then tip forward from the hip joints, let the head lead you up to high kneeling, one foot forward, maintaining balance between back and front foot, and continue your journey up to full standing.

Now go for a little 'directed' walk. Find your cardboard box, pick it up – remembering to pause and semiflex! – and place it on the floor a little distance from you. You'll notice that we have very hi-tech equipment in Alexander, and in a group you will have lots of boxes to play with. (Maybe I could patent Alexander cardboard boxes? Pilates have their balls, yoga their mats, Alexander their...?) All I want you to do now is walk forward and step in and out of the cardboard box(es), thinking up and out in a directed Alexander way. You do not have to get both feet into the box, just one will do, but next time you step in, use the other foot. At first you may be tempted to drop your neck to look down at the box, but of course by now you remember that it is possible to see 'down' in your peripheral vision and, if need be, change the angle of the eyeline by gently tipping the head from the top of your spine. I know, it's very Monty Python – I'm tricking you into being daft again! But not too much effort, is it? Now take yourself to the bottom of a handy nearby staircase. As you go to take the first step, pause and imagine instead that it's a box you are stepping into. Use this thought for every step on the staircase. Meet you at the top!

How was that? If you imagined this successfully, you will probably have found it a completely different experience, requiring much less effort than usual. My sister used to stamp up the stairs, making so much noise it drove me crazy. I taught her this cardboard-box trick and it completely changed the way she went upstairs. She was amazed. I am always amazed, too, at how such a little thought can effect such enormous change. If nothing shifted for you, keep playing – it may happen when you least expect it. Technically, what is happening is similar to marching on the spot. You are maintaining balance on one leg as the knee of the other leg goes up in front. We don't need to do that when we walk, but it is the action we use when we crawl, the knee sliding forward. So this is a 'vertical crawl'. Crawling upright, the support is on the back leg as the other leg steps into the box. It is also sabotaging the habitual length or contraction that your brain predicts you need when you look at the step. As you think of the foot dropping *into* rather than *onto* the step, you will be using momentum. What we so often do is to lean onto the bent front leg and heave ourselves up to full height from there. Bobbing up and down on one leg is a good strengthening exercise, something I use in the gym when I am prepping myself for my ten-kilometre run, but it's not what I need for simply walking upstairs.

Practise marching on the spot for a moment and then take your weight onto one leg, bending and straightening it a few times so you can experience the difference. If the stairs are deep, like the escalators on the London Underground (and I'm sure a lot of you have had the experience of having to walk up an out-of-action escalator), then you simply imagine a taller cardboard box, so the knee will come up higher.

Walking Downstairs

Going down the stairs, though, you need a different thought; the cardboard-box trick won't work. One idea is to remind yourself that it is the stairs going down, not you. You can maintain your 'up' direction. And the other accompanying thought is that the action is similar to crawling backwards in the upright. When you crawled backwards earlier, your head was leading and the lower leg slid away. So, as you walk down the stairs, keep the attention 'up' and allow the lower leg to extend away from the hip. By all means use the banister or wall to help your balance. If you are in a group, turn to watch everyone else as they walk down the stairs in this way. Walking with grace and elegance – are they about to receive their BAFTAs or Oscars, do you think?

Floating Fabulously

Knees Floating

Here's another way that can make going up stairs a little easier. In pairs have one lean against a wall and try to raise the knee. Your partner is stopping you, however, by pressing down on your leg. Maintain this conflict of interest for about fifteen seconds, then both give up the struggle, and now try raising the knee – wheeee! Up it comes! Do it with the other leg. Wheee! Now walk up the stairs. The knee automatically rises higher in marching mode. Swap. Soloists, play with this by facing a wall, almost touching it and try to take the knee forward and up, marching style. This time it is the wall creating resistance. Move away front the wall and try raising the knee again and you should get the same effect. So when you are about to walk up some stairs, pause, remember that effortless experience and ask for it back. You should find that you are directing yourself with ease.

This sense of floating is known as the Kohnstamm phenomenon and you are quite likely to have experienced it before when you were a kid. Ever stood in a doorway and tried to take your arms out to the side? Have a go now.

Arms Floating

First, take your arms up from your side and register the effort involved. Then stand in the doorway and try again to take your arms up. Do this for about fifteen seconds, then step away from the door frame and let the arms float up all on their own. Let the arms come down to your side again and, remembering that floating sensation, let them rise up again in a similar manner. Or you can do this in pairs. Have one of you stand or kneel behind the other and hold your partner's arms down at their side, restricting the upward movement as they try to raise them. After fifteen seconds, both of you stop the resistance and the arms of the one in front will float up easily. Again, experiment with taking the arms down and envisaging them floating up again. They will – perhaps not as much as before, but you will at least be starting from that place of effortless movement. If you want to learn more about this phenomenon there's plenty on the internet, along with results of the latest scientific trials. At present the exact reason for this phenomenon is still unknown, but it is definitely a neural function rather than a muscular one. Very Alexandrian!

Remember way back to Lesson One? In that first voyage into the nature of habits I suggested you could practise pausing before moving your arm to pick up a cup of tea, and redirect yourself by letting the hand lead the movement – more of a marionette movement than a lift and push forward from the shoulder. Have you been practising this? Here's another way to help with this cup-of-tea movement. Either in pairs or against a wall, restrict the forward and up movement of the arm for fifteen seconds and release in order to experience the Kohnstamm phenomenon again. Now, as you think of moving the arm towards your cup of tea – real or imaginary – pause and remember the floating sensation, and see if you can manage to recreate that as you take your hand forward.

If it is possible to restrict movement in our limbs and then find ease as we liberate them, isn't that perhaps what we are doing to the whole of ourselves as we inhibit our reactions and redirect our head, neck and back? We are not 'doing something', but taking away our habitual restrictions to discover lightness, ease and effortlessness.

A Voyage Around Your Arms

This experiment with our arms leads me neatly into considering more fully the upper limb. In this tour of our corporeal river, we have made forays into our head, neck, jaw, back, spine, pelvis, ribs, lungs, diaphragm, abdominals, legs and feet but, apart from casual observations, we have not yet meandered along the tributary of our upper limb.

We express ourselves so much through our arms. They are tender, sensitive, strong, flexible. We reach out with them to explore the world and we gather them in to protect us. They wave in the air to conjure images as we speak. As lovers we lie in each other's arms. They bring us close to each other so we can hear our hearts beat. They are intrinsically part of the whole of us and they connect us with others. They are not just a sticky-out bit that hangs like a salami sausage at our sides or stiffens to salute.

When we are mis-mapped, as you have realised by now, it can restrict our movement. So let's ask two key questions to explore your map. If we say the upper limb starts at the fingertips, where does it end? Where is the shoulder joint located? Spend a little while considering this. For yourself or in pairs discuss, poke yourself around, observe in a mirror and, as usual, check out what pictures and info you can find on the internet. Or you can just end-gain, cheat and continue reading!

The bones of the upper limb begin at the fingertips and finish where the collarbone meets the breastbone: the sternoclavicular joint is therefore the last joint of the arm.

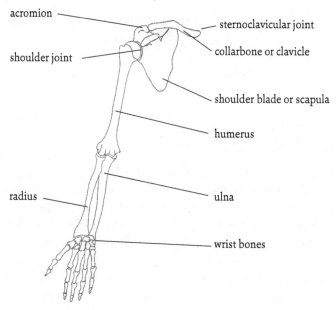

acromion

sternoclavicular joint

collarbone or clavicle

shoulder joint

shoulder blade or scapula

humerus

radius

ulna

wrist bones

The collarbone, or clavicle, is a wondrous little bone – often neglected – that enables us to shrug our shoulders or take our hand up over our head. It sits over the ribs, higher than the shoulder blades, attached to the acromion, and acts as a spreader bar to keep us open at the front. If a collarbone were to break, the shoulder blade would come forward as there is nothing to stop it. If we push our shoulder blades forward, the end of the collarbone has to rise to allow that movement.

The Moves of the Collarbone

Put the thumb of your right hand at the top of your breastbone and spread the rest of your fingers out to the end of your left collarbone. First shrug your shoulder then raise your arm above your head and you will feel the movement of the collarbone. Then push the shoulder blade forward and you will feel the collarbone squeeze itself forward and up. Study partners and groups, feel your partners' collarbones moving.

The shoulder blade sits below the collarbone has a rough triangular shape about the length of your hand and is not jointed to the ribs but embedded in muscle. It too is highly movable. It swings out from the base as we raise our arms, and swings forward as we take our arms forward.

The Moves of the Shoulder Blade

In pairs, have one partner place the flat of their hands on the other's shoulder blades and ask them to swing their arms up over the head and then to hug themselves. You will feel the shoulder blades disappear and then return home as they take their arms back again. Swap. Solo artists, have a go against the wall – at the very least you will feel lots of movement, but think through that movement as I described it and you may discern something more. Knowing that the last joint of the upper limb is the sternoclavicular may also make a difference to your movements. I invite you all to stand up for a moment and do a shoulder roll, as you would do often as part of a warm-up. Think of the movement starting from that joint at the top of your breastbone and think of the movement of your collarbone. After a few rolls one way, switch to the other. I suspect you will find that you experience the roll a little differently. Perhaps even a little easier?

Unlike the pelvic girdle, which needs to be firm and more fixed in place for support, the shoulder girdle is freely movable. The upper limb is not primarily for support but for movement, for manipulation and, originally, for hanging around in trees. This gives a clue as to where the muscles of the upper limb end. If you are suspended, you wouldn't want the leverage to end at the shoulder but to continue all the way down the back and across the front: the pecs, the traps, the lats – all arm muscles. As I mentioned in Lesson Three, the superficial muscles of the back are functionally arm muscles. Just pat yourself on the back for a moment. There you go, patting yourself on the upper limb again.

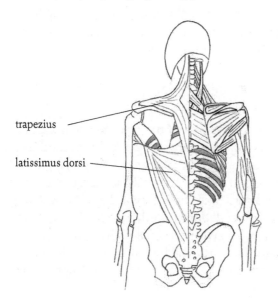

trapezius

latissimus dorsi

The trapezius, a diamond shape, starts at the occipital bone and covers the neck and shoulders, and extends longitudinally to the bottom of your thoracic vertebrae. The latissimus dorsi (Latin for 'widest back'), one of your back armpit muscles, attaches to the top of your arm, your mid to lower vertebrae and to the top of your pelvis. So we could say that the arm begins at the fingertips, goes up to the top of your neck, across to the spine and down to the top of your pelvis and the end of your sacrum.

Sensing the Lats

With your hand leading, take your arm forward and consider how that movement is coming all the way from the back. With partners, place your hands on the other's lower back and feel the muscles there move as your partner takes their arms forward or then above the head.

Other muscles that make up the whole muscularity of the upper limb at your back have beautiful names – terres major, terres minor, serratus anterior, the rhomboids, the deltoids, infraspinatus, supraspinatus... Google all of these arm muscles and you will see fabulous pictures of them.

Back to Back

Take it in turns to stroke the area of the trapezius and the area of the latissimus dorsi on your partner's back. Then stand back to back. Let's call you Apple and Pie. It works best if Apple and Pie are of a similar height. Apples, stay still and Pies, explore the movement of your arms. Take them forward and back, swing your arms above your head, both together, individually, to the side, and hug yourself. You will find you are giving your partner a very nice massage! The back will be warming up nicely, and how movable is that? Swap, so Pies stay still and Apples jive.

Soloists, lean into the wall and think of the muscles as you move your arms up and down and around – keep that picture of them in front of you if possible.

You've Got Some Front

At the front, the pectoralis muscles attach to the arm and shoulder and extend across to the collarbone, ribs and the length of the breastbone.

Feel the front armpit muscle – that's pectoralis major, one of the pecs. If you press the fingers of your right hand into your left armpit between the lat and the pec, you will be massaging the top and side of your ribs. The shoulder girdle sits over the ribs. When you shrug your shoulders, the whole shoulder girdle is sliding up and down your ribs. If you are not squeamish and your partner not ticklish, gently slide your fingers as far up as you can in your partner's armpit and you will be surprised how far in your fingers go, following the beehive shape of the ribcage.

We've Got Wings

Our pectoralis is the equivalent of a flight muscle in a bird. The breastbone would need to be sticking further forward by a few feet to enable us to flap our wings, of course, but you get the idea.

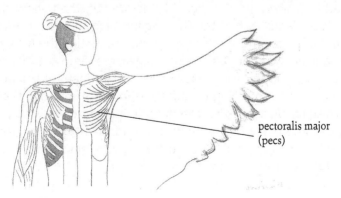

pectoralis major
(pecs)

Maybe your arms are already feeling a little bigger now you know they extend across the front of your ribcage and all the way down the back. Did you know your 'wingspan' is the same length as your height? That's enormous! Measure it to check it if you don't believe me! Open your arms out and, as you do so, think of them widening away from the breastbone. Thank goodness we have 'folds' in our arms, otherwise we would never get through doors. The arms fold and unfold. When you fold a piece of A4 paper, it doesn't get shorter, it's just folded. And can be folded back out to the same size. Same with our arms. These folds are at the finger joints, the wrist, the elbow, the shoulder, and the sternoclavicular, that new joint you've discovered where the collarbone meets the top of the breastbone. Let's remind the brain of the folds of your wings.

Spreading Your Wings

Lie in semi-supine with your arms spread out from your sides and, to centre yourself, consider your spatial direction both external and internal. Then gently raise your hands in the air, so they are hanging above the shoulders, arms subtly bent, very relaxed. You'll find it's bizarrely easy to balance them in this way. Remain in this position for a little while with palms turned towards each other, then point your fingers up to the ceiling and reach your arms up further so that you take your shoulder blades up off the floor. Stay like that for a few seconds, still breathing, nice and easy despite the stretch, then allow the shoulder blades to find the floor again, then the upper arms, then the lower arms and finally the hands, resting the back of the hand on the floor. Take them up again the same way: hands, lower arms, upper arms, pause to enjoy the natural balance, then point to the ceiling raising the shoulders and take them down again, bit by bit. Practise this a couple more times, so you can become really familiar with the folds in your wings. And when they rest at your side, you are likely to feel them longer, and the shoulders more relaxed and wider.

Enter the Shoulder Joint

Where did you think it was? Have a look at this picture and the shoulder joint as seen as part of the whole structure on page 217.

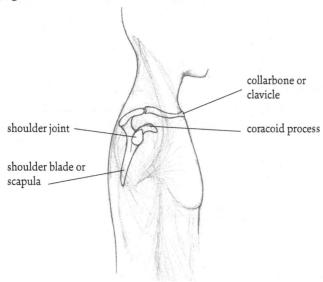

collarbone or clavicle

shoulder joint

coracoid process

shoulder blade or scapula

You will see that the joint itself is at the side and back, not at the front. One of our mis-maps places it like a raglan seam on a pullover. This mis-map leads us to pull our shoulders inwards and forwards, contracting our pectoralis muscles, narrowing our chest and creating a hunched look. We don't fly so well. This in turn interferes with the excursion of the ribs and therefore your breathing.

Finding the Shoulder Joint

Place your hand on the front of your chest and pull the shoulder forward. That's the shoulder girdle rotating best it can over your ribs. Very clunky. It's not using the shoulder joint at all. Now, leaving your shoulder alone, let your left arm hang down and cup your right hand at the top of your left arm. Turn your left arm in as far as it will go and turn it out as far as you will go. What you will feel is the rotation of the top of the humerus bone. Much more subtle and articulate! You are using your shoulder joint. If you explore with your fingers under the end of your collarbone – girls, where your bra strap often lies – you will perhaps find a nobbly lump. That is the front of your shoulder blade and it is called the coracoid process. The head of one of the biceps and the pectoralis minor attach there. Now see if you can find the gap between that nobbly bit and the head of the humerus, your upper arm bone. Got it? It's okay for there to be space between, it is not a joint and you will not dislocate it! The shoulder joint is further back. Place your thumb at the top of the breastbone, and your third and fourth fingers in the gap, directing towards the head of the humerus. There is the width of half your chest.

Placing the hand there and using your fingers in the gap to direct the humerus away from the shoulder blade can help your brain re-map the width of the chest and resite the shoulder joint. Check out more pictures of the shoulder joint on the internet. If you are in a pair or a group, have a poke around on someone else!

Here's something else you can play with to let your wings widen.

Widening Your Shoulders

In pairs, place the flat of your left hand at the front of your partner's left shoulder and the other hand at the back between the blade and the arm; direct your hands in towards each other and then slide them outwards and off the end of the left shoulder. Then repeat for the right shoulder. This is encouraging them to widen. Solo artists, find a partner to practise this on during the week if you can – and get them to do it to you. It's great!

Shoulders never have to be pulled back or squeezed forward. When left alone, they like to widen away from each other. Just for a moment, deliberately pull your shoulders back, hold them there and reach forward with your hands. You are immediately restricting the length of your reach. Now stop pulling them back and reach forward again. The shoulder can now respond to where your hand is going. Easier. I am not even going to put a question mark after that – it just is.

The following exercise uses the rotation of the arms to help enliven them and again widen the shoulders.

Rotating Your Arms

Stand with arms at your sides, palms forward, and turn the thumbs towards the body so the palms are backward, and then return them to where they were. Do this a few times.

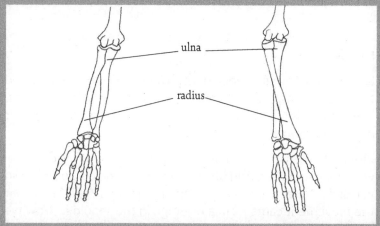

You will feel the lower arm rotating. The radius is rotating over the ulna which remains still. We use this rotation without thinking as soon as we have learned to balance our eggy weggy on the spoon, or turned our lower arm to touch the keyboard. Rotate the lower arm again, only this time continue to turn the thumb until you feel the upper arm join in. Turn a little further still so the palm is turned outwards, little finger to the front, and you will feel the shoulder girdle engage and come forward. Now rotate the other way, thumbs leading, until the palms are forward again. Continue the rotation outwards, and I think you will sense the upper arm and shoulder girdle rotating out, and your chest opening. Keep this opening stable for a moment and allow the thumb to turn only the lower arm back, the radius again turning over the ulna, palm back. Can you sense that the upper arm is still slightly away from your torso and the shoulder girdle still opening out? Allow the hands to float back to your side and you may still feel a lightness in the arms and that opening in the front of you.

You may be feeling very wide in the shoulders now after all the experiments and mapping. There's another exercise I want you to play with, that will also help release the shoulders and get the brain to recalibrate how the arm moves by giving the lead to the hand.

Flippers

Lie with your arms at your sides, hands palm-up. I've adapted this movement, called 'flippers', from the Dart Procedures, developed by Professor Raymond Dart, a devotee of Alexander's work.[3]

Move your left arm so that it is resting on the floor but level with your shoulder. And back again. How did you do that? Did you slide the arm, or pick it up and put it down? It is likely that the movement came from a leverage in the shoulder. Now we want your brain to change the movement of the arm by letting the hand lead and the rest follow. The signals, therefore, need to go to the hand first. So, keeping it palm up, simply deviate the hand, a sideways motion like a flipper, in the direction you want it to go, take the weight of the arm onto the fingertips, letting it rise up a little way from the floor, let the hand deviate again so it swivels the arm and then let it rest back on the floor. Do the same movement again and again – you will find that the whole arm is being flippered along the floor with the leverage in the hand, not the shoulder.

I sometimes imagine the hand as the head of a snake, exploring the world, and the rest of the arm snaking up after it. You can move your hand on the floor like this beyond the shoulder to above the head. Rest, and return it similarly to an easy place by your side. What seems a strange movement at first will suddenly become very easy. Try this with the other arm, and then both arms together. I think you will once again find that lovely connection all the way down your back to your pelvis, too.

You can also experiment with sensing how the thought precedes the action. Just think of doing one flipper, and then give up the idea. It is as though the arm fills itself and then empties itself of the thought. In the moment you give up the thought of moving it, move it. The arm will move, but perhaps with less effort. Great for practising inhibition!

A Wholesome Counterbalance

Arms are meant for reaching: mostly forward, sometimes to the side, but rarely to the back. Now you know the arms and shoulders are freely movable and do not require to be held. By releasing the arms you are no longer impinging on the action of the ribs so you are able to breathe better. They are also jolly useful for our balance. Ever balanced on a narrow beam or a plank? What happens instinctively? That's right – your arms come up to give you greater control of your balance. And when you take your arms forward, automatically the whole of the rest of you responds to that imbalance.

Arms Forward, Pelvis Back

Take your arms forward. What happens to the pelvis and the back? What is happening to the rest of you? If we are using our whole system, as the arms come forward, we counterbalance with all the body – the weight comes more to the back of the feet, and the pelvis swings back. If we are tightening the legs as we take the hands forward, we counterbalance by using the 'waist joint' to take our chest back, which means we are effectively leaning in the opposite direction, away from where we want our hand to go. Duhh! Do this movement several times – arms forward, bum back – until it feels easy. Does it remind you of something? Semiflexion, perhaps? This week, practise a wholesome counterbalance.

Staying in Touch

We know how to hold tight to the arms and how to collapse them, just as we did with the legs. But we will only be properly whole when we are doing neither of these things. Remapping will help us to include the arm within our sense of self, but as usual our psychophysical unity will manifest more easily when we widen our attention to the whole of us, as we have practised earlier in Lesson Two. We receive the world through the palm of our hand, our sensitive 'feeler', so let's make the hand the portal, that part of us from which we start to widen our attention. We can use either our spatial awareness or the directions of the earth supporting us up through our bony structure.

Just the Touch of Your Hand

In pairs, have one place their hand on the partner's shoulder. Brace the arm and then collapse the arm. Partner give instant feedback as to the quality of their touch. You will feel it too – that you are pushing them away as you brace your arm and inadvertently pulling them towards you when you collapse the arm. Your partner will also tell you how heavy it feels! So do neither. Do not brace nor collapse, but stay in touch. Give attention to the three-dimensional quality of the hand, the space it takes up, and pass that thought on to the whole arm, the torso, the neck and shoulders, the head, and down to the legs, until you are experiencing your whole self as a three-dimensional space. Different? Swap and discuss. Solo players, you can easily do the same with the wall. Place your hand on the wall, bracing the arm and then collapsing it. In the latter instance the arm will slip down the wall to your side. But the next time choose to keep the hand on the wall and change your awareness to the three-dimensional space you are taking up, starting from the hand, and then include more and more of you in your awareness. The wall will be supporting you in a very different way.

Now place the other hand on the wall or your partner's shoulder. Brace and collapse the arm as before, then find the middle ground where you are just in touch. This time experiment with the 'up' direction that the contact force of the earth is lending you through the wall or through your partner. Direct the wrist away from the fingertips, the elbow away from the wrist, the shoulder away from the elbow, the back away from the shoulder, the neck freeing, the head rising up, the knees lengthening out of the hip joints, the ankles out of the knees, the feet dropping out of the ankles, spreading onto the floor. Different again? Swap and discuss. Both are valid, but you may prefer one to the other.

As you become aware of your whole self, the touch will not be collapsed or braced but lightly responsive, reaching out to the world and receiving the world, the whole of you touching the whole of them, responding to your fellow actor, neither pushing them away nor pulling them towards you. And when we are whole, those awkward moments onstage when your hands feel enormous (and thank goodness you've got pockets to shove them in), will go. I once played Professor Higgins in a school production and oh my, did my hands feel like something from *Alice in Wonderland*, growing bigger and bigger by the second! But as we allow ourselves to become whole, the arms won't feel like separate, heavy bits that have to be held up. In fact they will cease to exist as sticky-out bits – you will be, as it were, pretty 'armless.

Standing and Sitting

So now you are fully cognisant regarding arms. You have some great experiments to help release those shoulders, and you know how arms can either be separate salami sausages or represent the responsive wholeness of you. You know how to walk up and down stairs gracefully, have experienced the Kohnstamm phenomenon to help your ease of movement and balance, and sung 'Summertime' out of tune. Can there be anything more to consider? You can walk tall, sit well, stand easy... but do you move easily from sitting to standing, and from standing to sitting?

Let's explore that journey, a movement we are making all the time and rarely think about. Our whole system is rebalancing itself, going from two legs to six legs (if it's a four-legged chair), six legs to two legs. What is your personal choreography?

Experiments in Standing and Sitting

Use a mirror or film yourself, or work in pairs. Have one of you stand and sit a few times, whilst the other observes your pattern of movement, then discuss and swap. (I bet you are getting more accurate in your observations now.) You may notice how we use our arms in this acrobatic feat, often pushing ourselves off the chair, or swinging the arms forward or hunching our shoulders up. And what's happening with the breath? We often hold our breath during this action. Is your neck tightening, head tipping back and your spine arching and shortening?

Apart from the choreography, what effort are you using to stand and sit? Using all the tools we have worked with so far, can you devise a way to make it easier? Play with this idea for a moment. Inhibit and direct yourself. Do not try hard: we can all sit and stand, it's fairly easy. You are just practising finding new ways of doing things in a non-doing way!

Here are some ideas that might help:

- Don't think that in order to sit you have to 'go down'. You exist all the way down to your feet, and they are not going down. Your knees are going forward, they are not going down. Your head and torso are definitely lowering in space, but you are simply changing shape and changing your balance. Think 'up' before you begin the movement.

- You have already discovered that it is easier on our system if we can balance forward. If you balance backwards to sit, the only way of remaining balanced is by contracting a whole lot of muscles, and this adds tension, particularly in the back. Instead, balance forward from the ankles and send the knees forward. You'll soon realise that sitting is an up and over direction, not back and down.

- Notice how you are going through semiflexion in both directions (we are in semiflexion most of the time!). Remember the experiments with pausing and changing the thought of which direction you were going in? Does it help now in sitting?

- Place a hand at the back of your neck (or your partner's, if you're in pairs) and, as you stand or sit, try to avoid squashing the fingers together. This will prevent the head being pulled back and keep the neck long; the top of your spine will be lengthening and you can maintain that length throughout the torso. Think: 'Neck free; let the head go forward and up; let the back lengthen and widen.'

- Inhibit the desire to pull your chest up as you stand and, instead, rock forward on your sitting bones, find your feet beneath you, and let the top and back of your head lead you up to standing. The head leads and the spine follows, legs unfolding.

- Think of the upthrust of the earth through your bones still taking you up, even as you sit, and hitch a ride on that force as you stand.

- Think of yourself as a marionette, everything folding and unfolding as your head moves through space.

- Instead of sitting and standing facing forward from the chair, turn your head and spiral upwards so you end up standing by the side of the chair, facing the other way. Can you do that in reverse, so you spiral down to the chair?

- Take one foot back as you go to stand or sit.

- Direct your attention away from the choreography altogether and focus on the space and environment around you. Be aware of the distance between the top of your head and the ceiling; the distance between your back and the wall behind; the space between you and whatever is in front, and note how those spatial parameters change as you come from sitting to standing.

- Is there any way you could use the Kohnstamm phenomenon?

Which of these was the easiest for you? Discuss, or jot down your findings in your logbook.

In individual lessons, an Alexander teacher will often use sitting and standing to help you discover the nature of your habits and ways of changing them through inhibition and direction. Alexander used this as a main activity too and whilst it is crucial for you as an actor to be effortless in your uprising and your alighting (I love that an alternative word to sitting has the syllable 'light' in it!), be warned by the man himself:

'Boiled down, it all comes down to inhibiting a particular reaction to a given stimulus. But no one will see it that way. They will see it as getting in and out of the chair the right way. It is nothing of the kind. It is that a pupil decides what he will or will not consent to do.'[4]

'It's not getting in and out of chairs, even under the best of conditions, that is of any value; that is simply physical culture – it is what you have been doing in preparation that counts when it comes to making movements.'[5]

Happy movement-making this week!

Assignments

- Lie down in semi-supine and practise moving your arms in segments up above your shoulders and balancing them there before taking them back to the floor. Play *Flippers*.

- Stick up some pictures of arm bones and muscles, or change the wallpaper on your devices from breathing apparatus to the arms.

- Stand with arms at your sides and experiment with the rotations.

- Let your hand lead your movements.

- Practise counterbalancing as you take your hands forward.

- When you touch the wall, a piece of furniture, even another person, be aware of how the touch is being directed – not collapsed or braced – and use it to come into a sense of the whole self.

- Inhibit when going up and down stairs, and think of cardboard boxes and crawling backwards for an easier experience!

- Have fun with the Kohnstamm phenomenon and use it as a direction after inhibiting the initial stimulus.

- Experiment with sitting and standing. Because we do this all day long, thinking of it consciously every time is a tall order, so perhaps choose a particular room, chair or situation to practise with, in the same way we chose cleaning our teeth as practice for semiflexion. Inhibit, direct, attention up and out, responsive – head will be leading.

Lesson Ten: The Transformational Vortex and Other Acting Fun

Applying the work to characterisation and performance

Equipment

- A wall

- A favourite piece of dance music and something to play it on

- Space to dance wildly and walk around in

- A chair

- If in a group, a copy of 'The Moon Like a Bone in the Sky: A Happening' from Appendix C, with instructions cut out and distributed as indicated (see page 245)

'God guard me from the thoughts men think
In the mind alone;
He that sings a lasting song
Thinks in a marrow-bone'

W. B. Yeats[1]

How was your week? Check in with study partners and/or your logbook. As usual, there was quite a lot to play with: allowing the huge wings that cover your torso to fold and unfold, rotate and flip; playing with the Kohnstamm phenomenon to help you inhibit and direct; stepping into cardboard boxes instead of going up stairs; and continuing awareness of semiflexion as you sit and stand.

A Recitation on the Move

Remember this nursery rhyme?

'Mary had a little lamb,
Its fleece was white as snow,
And everywhere that Mary went
The lamb was sure to go.'

Recite this as you slide up and down a wall; recite it as you semiflex; recite it as you sit and stand. The use pattern is the same – one is vertical, one is tipping the torso forward; one uses the wall for support, one uses a chair. But the breath and vocal mechanisms are not interfered with, whatever the movement. Get it?

This exercise employs fairly formal movement, obeying the laws of our structure to find easy mobility and balance.

Today let's get some jive going, applying this work to help you transform into another character. Let's think about taking Alexander Technique into performance and see how it can help with nerves.

Inhabiting the Use of a Character

Musical Statues

Get the music going, let your hair down and dance, girl/guy! If Alexander can give you effortless movement, let's see some. Go wild – abandon yourself to the music – yay! Then suddenly stop, as you might do in a game of musical statues, holding the position. Stand in that position and, without making any effort to change, just think your directions – spatial or internal lengthening and widening ones – releasing yourself into the shape you found yourself in but letting go of any excessive tension you may have been using to maintain the pose. After releasing into that shape, dance madly again! And freeze again – release again. As you maintain that released shape, walk the shape around, taking in the world. Return to your dance spot, continuing to think of the expansive directions, and then allow your head to come up and let the rest follow. You are using this releasing movement to come back to a centred balance. Try that once again – dance wildly, freeze, release but keep the shape, walk the shape around, back to your dance spot, then continue the expansive release, head leading to bring you back to a restored neutral balance.

What do you reckon? Can you sense that in this way you can maintain any shape you need for a character without having to give yourself backache and vocal tension? Make a fist with your hand, and now release the tension from it whilst keeping the shape. Easy, isn't it? Just the right amount of effort. Then allow the whole fist to unfold so your hand is open and relaxed.

Imagine you were playing Richard III, or Laura from *The Glass Menagerie*, every night. These characters have specific shapes and use, which you, as the actor, are inhabiting organically, and in this way you can inhibit any excessive tension involved and you'll also be able to release yourself from the shape after the curtain comes down or the cameras have stopped rolling. I love that 'end of play' moment when the cast come onstage for the curtain call and the actors can lay their characters aside, walking and breathing as themselves once more.

I hope you don't think that I am suggesting that in order to be a great actor you need to maintain an Alexandroid symmetry in everything you do – the 'cardboard box on two legs' thing. No, that would not help you transform at all. We are movable beings, flexible, changeable and responsive, and as actors you are giving yourselves the option of choosing from an immense palette of movement and voice in order to portray a living soul onstage and on-screen. You are removing the limitations of your habit, that's all, finding an Alexander 'centre' from which you can transform.

If you are working in a group, you can actually play musical statues the old way first off, just for fun. Have someone turn the music off suddenly from time to time and eliminate anyone who moves after the music has stopped. Competition and elimination are exciting and also highlight how hard we try to win, and what tension we employ! I suspect there will be a lot of you holding your breath, or breathing shallowly. When you've played a round of that, go through the Alexander experiment as previously outlined.

> 'When an investigation comes to be made, it will be found that every single thing we are doing in the Work is exactly what is being done in nature where the conditions are right, the difference being that we are learning to do it consciously.' F. M. Alexander[2]

Although you will want to be the shape appropriate to your role, I would suggest, as you begin your Alexander journey, that it's often good to make decisions about a character's movement patterns that avoid your own habit. For example, if you have a habit of slumping and pulling down, you may feel intuitively that a character who is shy and nervous should have a similar use. Challenge that notion. Allow yourself to be at full height and experience how dreadful it is if you are shy and yet stick out like a sore thumb. If you are someone who braces themselves up, holds the legs and sticks the chest out, and you are playing a flirtatious sort – well, maybe there is another, more sinuous way. You are already experts in your own habits and you don't need to practise them any more. It's much more interesting to venture into unfamiliar territory.

The Transformational Vortex[3]

Here's an exercise to help you transform your own use patterns into that of someone else. Stand easy for a moment and think of someone you know well, but not a member of your family. If you are doing this in a group or in pairs, make sure it is someone outside of the Alexander/theatre world, so that your peers will not recognise the individual. As you think of this person, allow yourself to take on their body shape and their use pattern, and walk around the room. Solo artists, please film yourself doing this and then review it. In pairs, take it in turns to perform this in front of your partner. In groups, do it one at a time in front of the rest.

Study partner or group, as the individual walks round, consider what character you see taking shape before you. Call out your best guess for gender, age, type of work, personality, family situation, leisure activities. Actor, please play the fourth wall and don't comment until they have said as much as they want. Then stop walking in character, tell them the name of the person and discuss what they'd got right. This can be surprisingly accurate, showing how much is conveyed just by body shape and the way someone moves. Solo artists, having looked back at yourself on film walking as the Person You Know Well, film yourself walking around the room again but this time as yourself. Looking back at this film, do you notice the difference? Can see yourself as a stranger? And what would you make of this person who is walking around? Do they look confident, happy, intense? Do they look as if they'd be good with children? Would they be sitting behind a desk all day? Whatever you perceive about yourself from an objective point of view. Inhibit your familiarity with your known self!

Study partner or group, give this 'character', the actor, the same treatment as before – you can probably see gender and age, but pretend for a moment that you know nothing about them. What is suggested by the way they are walking – the type of work they do, their personality? This can be an eye-opener for the actor, and it might give some idea of future casting. It goes without saying that it is always a supportive subjective analysis! Read through the following carefully first and then try it out. If you are in a group or with a partner it may help if someone prompts the actor by reading or improvising around the paragraph below. In this case, use their real name, rather than 'Base Character', and the real name of their friend, rather than Person you Know Well.

Now, actor, draw an invisible circle on the floor. This is your Transformational Vortex. Step into this circle and just as you stopped being the Person You Know Well, stop being Who You Think You Are – we'll call this 'Base Character' (BC) – and allow your Inner Actor, or the Higher Creative Self, to emerge. Higher Creative Self has been playing the role of Base Character for a long time – twenty years or more? – so right now she/he can have a rest and let go of the Base Character's history, emotions, beliefs, hopes and aspirations. I guess the only emotion Higher Creative Self may have right now is wonder and curiosity. Higher Creative Self honours Base Character and all she/he has been through and, as Base Character leaves, she/he manifests beside you on your left. You can drop back into being her/him again any time you want. But just for now, perhaps it's possible to let your Base Character go. It may be that BC liked to hold on to the legs a little, or hold her/himself down, but as Higher Creative Self you don't have to do that any more. And, no longer limited by memory, you can look up and about the room with curiosity. It may be a space that BC is very familiar with, but Higher Creative Self has never seen it through her/his own eyes before, so feel free to walk about the space, exploring those strange shapes that are called chairs, or the unknown white things stuck to the wall that click when you touch them and make light overhead. You can have a ball walking through the room and exploring BC's world for the first time, noticing also how easy it is to move now you are no longer stuck in the patterns of BC but can walk as yourself.

When you are ready, Higher Creative Self, return to the Transformational Vortex, and notice that to your right the character of the Person Base Character Knows Well is manifesting. Since you can become anyone, do anything and are no longer bound by the constraints of BC, drop into being the Person Base Character Knows Well and take her or him for a walk. When you are ready, come back to the Transformational Vortex and let go of Person Base Character Knows Well, enjoying being unencumbered by their use patterns. Notice that on the left is your old familiar Base Character and gently, slowly allow yourself to drop back in to being her/him again. You may feel quite a shift. Soloists, please watch the film back and compare the manifestations of BC, Higher Creative Self and the two versions of Person You Know Well. Groups and study partners, please discuss your experiences and your observations.

Whatever you experienced or observed is entirely valid. Each person's journey will be different. Some may not find it so easy to let go of their defined character or personality and inhabit the creative space. For others it can be a deep transformational experience. I have known some people who have not wanted to return to their old selves, having enjoyed at last the liberation of Higher Creative Self. Some are so moved and have travelled so far that they are unable to put their experience into words. As actors, when you fully inhabit the world of the drama you are creating new neural networks; changing your brain.

If there is time, group members can take it in turn to play with this one, or you can do a whole group experiment. Having seen it demonstrated by one person, have a go with all of you doing it together, drawing your own Transformational Vortices and stepping inside. Or you could divide the group so that half watches, half takes the exercise. It is an unvoiced exercise. The Creative Self, or the Inner Actor, are terms I heard used in Michael Chekhov's work,[4] a way of accessing the unconscious creative self through movement, gesture and intuition. I added the term 'Higher' to suggest that 'up' direction and our ability to perceive things from a higher perspective. Making it a non-verbal exercise helps it to stay intuitive, beyond the word-based intellect. Many respond that when the Higher Creative Self inhabits the Person You Know Well, the depiction becomes fluid, believable and truthful, not just an imitation of a movement, as we saw in the first walkabout. Then the actor was going straight from habit-based self to the character. The second time, they lose themselves and let Higher Creative Self do the acting. Higher Creative Self tends to be anarchic, like a child, a white-faced clown, without ego or constraint. We couldn't live in this state for long and still get on in the world, but we can choose to inhabit it more often. I think it is an effortless state of being we access in Alexander Technique. And the journey between the old, habitual self and the up, open, responsive, easy self becomes shorter and easier to access. Sometimes when we start Alexander work we think we need to be in the Hotel of Good Use, which is up the road out of sight, whilst we are grovelling around in the Hovel of Misuse.[5] What we are after is the road between the two, the means whereby we can change

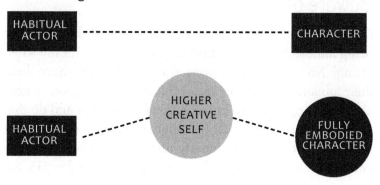

It might be fun to go on and explore vocalising Higher Creative Self. Does she/he have a different voice? Do they express themselves in words or just sounds? As soon as we start vocalising, our intellect is tempted to start up again, so watch out for that. I leave that one for you to play with and develop.

You can use this method to help you in text work and rehearsal. The Person BC Knows Well could be the character you are rehearsing and you can use *The Transformational Vortex* as a way of finding your character before you go into the scene. Higher Creative Self has no concerns or shame. She/he lives in the moment and doesn't worry about consequences. If you get embarrassed singing, for example, just step into your vortex, let go of your Base Character and let Higher Creative Self take over for a moment. Or think of a wonderful, confident singer you know and, via Higher Creative Self, drop into being that person. This is an extraordinary, powerful tool.

I hope this has quashed any ideas that Alexander Technique is simply something to help your posture. It is a psychophysical discipline, a tool to help you inhabit a creative space unencumbered by habits that restrict you. Remember Michelangelo releasing the angel from the block of marble? We are chipping away at the old habits, the old patterns of use, to reveal the Inner Actor or Higher Creative Self within.

Beware of Thinking!

Do you have to think of Alexander Technique whilst onstage or being filmed? No. Do you think of your voice specifically when acting? No – the voice classes and your practice have done their job and you are 'on voice'. But if you were given a note about walking to a certain mark, you'll remember and do that even whilst in character. Or you might be told at a certain point that you can't be heard properly, and therefore you'll practise and remember this when that point comes round again. So, similarly, if you are told you are looking crunched up, tense and inappropriate, you can respond to this. One MA student I worked with was a fabulous actor, very watchable, and yet in his second project seemed not to be onstage at all. What had happened? I discovered he was experimenting with thinking about his directions and use. His attention had narrowed: he was no longer present and responsive. When I watch great acting I am never conscious of the actor's use because it merges seamlessly with who they are, a fully embodied, responsive whole. If I'm only aware of their neck sticking forward every time they speak, they are not transformed or inhabiting the role fully, and it becomes a conflicted performance. However, to train yourself to associate being out of habit onstage, here's an exercise you can play with from time to time.

Acting 'Up'

The most important thing is that, whatever the instruction or script, you are to maintain a healthy, neutral 'up', responsive and balanced Alexander state. That is key. Now, solo artist and pairs practise these simple instructions, memorise them, and then film them.

Walk over to the chair, sit and wait for someone else to join you. After a count of ten, look round to see where they are for a count of ten. Then look back, sit still and wait for another count of ten. Then look at your watch for a count of ten. Hear a sound, and look round again for a count of ten. Then look back, sit still and wait for a count of ten. Repeat that sequence. Next time do the same sequence, but instead of just turning your head to look round, get up from the chair to turn round and look, and then sit back. Repeat this sequence. For the third sequence, stand up, turn round and call out 'Hello?' Repeat this sequence. Then stay still, looking forward, and choose in the moment an action, for example: check your mobile, or lean back and fold your arms, mutter under your breath, do a tap dance! And then, whenever you choose, end the action by walking away. Groups, use 'The Moon Like a Bone in the Sky: A Happening' (see Appendix C on page 279). You will each have different instructions. Let it unfold as it will. When you've finished filming, play it back and watch carefully. As in the solo performance above, they are just simple actions, devoid of character or 'inner life', which means you can keep your attention out and be in an Alexandrian state – even if the instruction is for you to cry like a baby! It's great fun to play with, as you won't know what is going to happen or what anyone else is doing. Very in-the-moment. As you watch it back, are you doing what you thought you were doing? Are you maintaining that Alexander centre?

Sometimes people will say 'I don't need to practise this coming-out-of-habit malarkey – I can assume it when I am onstage.' Hmmm, maybe. But you may find that, despite your best endeavours to maintain that initial instruction, you will get caught up in the action and forget the Alexander direction altogether.

Remember, this is just an exercise to practise Alexander thinking whilst acting, instead of practising whilst cleaning your teeth or getting up from a chair. It's great to practise whilst you are doing a Meisner repetition exercise, too.[6] Meisner is very compatible with Alexander because it is asking you to take the attention outside of yourself and respond in the moment, according to the stimulus given, the conditions and the stakes. If you are not familiar with Meisner's repetition exercises, here is my simple beginner's version – please have a go at this right now.

A Meisner Repetition Exercise

Stand in pairs, facing each other. One person notices something about the other and tells what they notice, e.g. 'You are wearing a red dress.' The partner replies by repeating the statement but swapping the pronoun, e.g. 'I am wearing a red dress.' This continues until one of the pair notices something else and changes the statement accordingly, e.g. 'You are blinking.' / 'I am blinking.' 'You are blinking.' / 'I am blinking.' 'You are smiling.' / 'I am smiling.' 'You are frowning.', etc. If you are working alone, you can do this with your reflection in the mirror or the image on screen. Of course, you will have to voice the reflection's repetition and the change will always come from you – an interesting identity crisis! But I promise it does still work. It doesn't matter if you pause. 'You're not saying anything.' / 'I'm not saying anything.' 'You're speaking a lot.' / 'I'm speaking a lot...' There will always be something to be observed and commented on. Just remember to start the process by commenting on the other person, or the reflection, your image on the screen, not yourself.

This links in with a previous experiment in Lesson Two, where I suggested you practise occupying the chattering mind by talking through what you can see, hear, feel or are doing, in order to become present. This time the focus is on the other person as part of the environment. Make sure you don't narrow your focus. Still keep that healthy widened attention even though you are connecting and commenting on your partner or reflection or screen image. As we use different neural pathways for our balance, our brain opens up to other unknown, unconsidered territories. It's an indirect way of finding that creative space again, a new neural network. Like finding Higher Creative Self.

Using the Vortex for Meisner

Higher Creative Self is very good at Meisner repetition. Once you have practised *A Meisner Repetition Exercise* as described, draw that invisible circle on the floor, let go of Base Character to release Higher Creative Self, and have another go. Please make notes in your logbook, and/or discuss with study partners how all these acting and Alexander exercises have worked for you.

Lights, Action...

So there you are: already primed, on voice, limbered up, Alexandered out, and the camera is about to roll or the lights come up. What's your state, as you are waiting to begin? Nervous? Or excited? Bit of both? The same chemical processes apply in both states, it's how we interpret them that is key. We need a little adrenalin to give us a heightened consciousness and energy for performance. You wouldn't be standing, chilled out, at the start of a running track and only spring into life once the starter pistol goes. No, we need a little prep: 'Readiness is all', as Alexander was fond of quoting from *Hamlet*.[7] It's okay to have butterflies, but you may want them to fly in formation, as various gurus – including Michael Gelb, Alexander teacher, and public speaker[8] – suggest. (Just imagining those beautiful winged creatures forming a victory 'V' in my belly always made me feel good and changed my state.) However, sometimes we get overanxious and, despite all the prepping, we are a bunch of nerves. A lot of fright and anxiety comes from our habit of imagining the worst. Remember that experiment with the five-finger piano exercise in Lesson Two? Going through the exercise in the head was almost as good practice as the real thing. Similarly, one way of overcoming that habitual dread is to practise being calm and confident by going through the whole performance in your mind, imagining yourself to be doing it brilliantly, just as you would want. See it, hear it, taste it, smell it, be in touch with it – and hear the applause at the end, or the director saying, 'Thank you, that's a wrap – just what we wanted. Excellent performance.' When the UK athlete Sally Gunnell was in the final for the women's 400m hurdles in the 1993 World Championships in Stuttgart, she had a horrible cold. She concealed it from her fellow athletes, and thought only of being well and running well. She broke the world record. You've practised this in a small way before, by imagining yourself rolling over from lying down in semi-supine to coming to standing easily, so you are already familiar with this skill of imagining your future going really well. So now, in your imagination, give yourself the joy of performing well. Then, when you then step into the lights, or the camera starts rolling, you are stepping into and living a future you have already created for yourself.

But my feeling is that if you are following all the principles of Alexander – inhibiting your immediate reaction, directing yourself, heeding your primary control, widening your attention, being spatially aware, using yourself effortlessly with gravity, not end-gaining but staying present, allowing the world to come to you, lying in semi-supine regularly, sitting well, walking tall, breathing easily, balancing freely – then those nerves just might take a back seat anyway. Although I didn't realise it, I always looked a little glum as I walked down the street deep in thought in my inner world. Of course, wretched builders (why was it always them?) would feel perfectly at liberty to tell me to 'Cheer up, love, it may never happen!' My hackles would go up, and inward seething – if not explosive retorts – would follow. However, as I began to work with Alexander, I realised after a while that all those comments had stopped. I hadn't tried to stop looking glum or feeling miserable, but my experience of Alexander, my change of use, indirectly changed something I hadn't directly considered.

The Dressing-up Box

There's one more thing I want to set up for you as a transforming experience. Remember your love of the dressing-up box?

Changing Your Clothes

Just think about the clothes you are wearing now and the clothes you usually wear. Sometimes it will depend on what you're doing – rehearsal blacks? – but there may be a style that you favour. Perhaps you don't ever wear orange, or only like loose-fitting clothes, trendy trainers, plain colours not patterns or frills, and certainly you wouldn't ever be caught dead in a suit and tie, twin-set or faux fur. Jot down in your logbook the things you would rarely wear, along with other habits regarding your appearance or how you present yourself. Do you wear your hair straight, never use gel, wash it every day? Earrings but no necklace; a watch, make-up? Do you always make sure you are looking neat and tidy, or prefer a slightly ruffled look? Clean-shaven or stubble? Jot it all down and discuss with your study partners. Isn't it interesting that, consciously or unconsciously, we all create a 'look' for ourselves. Trendy, sporty, goth, chav, nice, casual, smart, conservative, alternative, arty… First we wear what our parents put us in, and then at some point we are influenced by our own tastes and by fashion trends. So (you know what I am going to suggest) have a think about how you could change this habit or get your study partners to suggest what you could wear in order to change your appearance for a day.

Nothing ridiculous, or inappropriate for the season. Don't spend a lot of money on this – beg steal or borrow – and don't shave off your beard if you are in a Chekhov at the moment, but have some fun and challenge yourself. Choose not to wear make-up if you usually do, put on some lippy if you never do, try not washing your hair, try out heels or flats, the tight red T-shirt, the revealing blouse, the baggy trousers, the sloppy pullover, Y-fronts or boxers, bra or braless, etc. Select a day when it will be easy for you to change appearance. Go out publicly in your changed attire, even if it's just to walk down the road or get on a bus. Even better, though, meet with family or friends so you can get feedback. Have they noticed? Will they say anything? If you're working as a group or in partners, choose next week's Alexander lesson as your day of change, so that you can enjoy seeing everyone else dressed unusually, and give each other feedback.

One acting student, who often wore formal clothes, discovered how playful he felt when he was wearing a hoodie and jeans. A serious young student, who always wore black, discovered how fabulous and warm she looked wearing deep, rich colours. Her eyes shone! She saw another side to herself. Her clothes changed how she was feeling. This is what many great actors do to help them find their character: first find the costume. I believe the actor Beryl Reid would decide on the character's shoes first, and wear them right from very early on in rehearsal. On the other hand, it may not be a very comfortable experience at all. An acting student who always wore a fringe with lots of make-up, accessories and sparkles, arrived the following week in a pleated skirt, no make-up, hair tied back. I have never seen anyone look so miserable in my whole life. Then there was the guy who always wore loose-fitting, scruffy grey clothes and arrived for the day in a bright, tight-fitting shirt and bum-hugging trousers, hair shorn and red-framed glasses – totally transformed and, may I say on behalf of all of us in the room, looking 'up', alert and gorgeous. But he wouldn't believe it, didn't like it, and the very next day reverted to his more comfortable 'look'. How powerful appearance can be in how we feel about ourselves, how we use ourselves, and how others perceive us.

I used to love this exercise – once a year at the drama school I could stop looking like an Alexander teacher (flat shoes, clothes I can move easily in, no make-up, long loose hair, alternative and purple maybe), and arrive at school wearing either a glamorous, short red dress, with frizzy hair and the highest of heels; or my 'scary headmistress' look, with a formal skirt and jacket, and hair scraped back in a French pleat. On these days I was always made-up and often had tons of jewellery, frills and swirly patterns – yuck! I confess I only wore those heels for the effect of walking in the door, and kicked them off very quickly. I would find myself holding my hands differently, as if presenting my fingers to show them covered in nail varnish, and I could feel my face beginning to freeze if I were in jacket and skirt, my shoulders tightening when I wore a thin turtle-neck sweater.

Our clothes can affect our use. When you go up for casting, it goes without saying that you could lean towards how you think that role should look. But now it's time to play. When we change our appearance just for fun, it's like the Hawthorne Effect I wrote about before. It interrupts our routine; we pay attention, and our energy goes up. We can transform by letting go of our character and by letting go of our clothes!

'What a piece of work is a man! How noble in reason, how infinite in faculty, in form and moving, how express and admirable, in action how like an angel, in apprehension how like a god! The beauty of the world, the paragon of animals!' William Shakespeare[9]

Assignments

- Lie down in semi-supine. Use the time to practise imagining a future performance going really well.

- Practise changing your use by noting the shape you are in; release the tension from the shape and let your head lead you 'up' to a more conducive standing or sitting balance.

- Practise letting go of your habitual self, your Base Character, and allow Higher Creative Self to come out to play.

- Change your appearance for a day.

'Talk about a man's individuality and character: it's the way he uses himself.' F. M. Alexander[10]

Lesson Eleven:
That's a Wrap!
Time for the
After-show Party...

Reviewing and assessing how far you've come and where to go from here

Equipment

- Filming equipment
- The film you made of yourself in Lesson One
- A chair
- A piece of A4 paper
- Coloured pens
- The picture you drew of yourself in Lesson One
- Baroque music and a sweetie
- Your logbook

'People say that what we're all seeking is a meaning for life. I don't think that's what we're really seeking. I think that what we're seeking is an experience of being alive, so that our life experiences on the purely physical plane will have resonances with our own innermost being and reality, so that we actually feel the rapture of being alive.'
Joseph Campbell[1]

How was your week? What's it like to wear different clothes? How was lying down? Anything come up from acting experiences? Have you played with Higher Creative Self? Any thoughts or observations you have had, please share now with your study partners or check out your logbook and reflect. If you are in a group, remember it is useful to start talking in twos before sharing with the wider group, otherwise it might be always the same spokespeople opening up whilst others listen. By talking about what we have learned, we remember it more strongly.

The Review

Let's repeat the experiment in Lesson Three when you first played with Alexander Technique.

Directing Yourself Again

Stand and speak a few lines of text aloud. Then stand in the Alexander way, directing yourself and, instead of speaking, do nothing. Next time you think of speaking the text, walk backwards instead. Then, as you think of speaking the text, make a choice: you can speak, walk backwards or just stand there and take no action other than to keep your directions going. Play with this a few times, sometimes speaking, sometimes walking backwards, sometimes taking no action but to stand there. Next time, think of speaking the text but do nothing; give yourself the option of walking backwards, and then speak the text. Play with that a few times. The response to the stimulus to speak is delayed for a moment as you make a conscious choice not to speak; to have the option of walking backwards but, in the end, choosing to speak. Is this feeling more familiar? Is it making more sense to you? Feel free to organise this as a group event as before.

Having done that, let's repeat the filming you did in Lesson One, when you first looked at your habitual use patterns. This is a sort of repeat, but the difference is that now I hope you will be using yourself consciously, making choices about how you do these simple actions; directing yourself. Maybe you will be using semiflexion as you pick something up; being aware of the space around you as you stand; using the travelator to walk to the back of the room and back; staying in an easy balance with wide, inclusive attention as you speak and sing.

Filming Yourself Again

Set up the equipment as before, so that all of you can be seen, not just head and shoulders. Place a chair in the middle of the space, sideways to camera so you can be seen in profile. Choose a line or two of text as before – either the same as in Lesson One or something new – and a line or two from a song. ('Summertime'?) Stand away from the camera or screen, so you can be seen in full figure and – PAUSE! INHIBIT, DIRECT – and say, 'Hi, my name is… and I am going to speak a line of text from… and sing a line from…' Then stand in front of the chair, sit and stand twice in profile, turn away from the camera and walk away to the back of the room. Walk back towards the chair, and turn again in profile, just as you were standing before. Pick up something imaginary from the floor and place it on an imaginary high shelf. Then speak your line of text and sing your line of song, remaining in profile to the camera. If you are working in a group or in pairs, have one stand there and introduce the other and their lines of text and song. And do applaud when they have finished.

Bravo! Film over. Wait for it! Do not look back at it yet. Do not end-gain! Instead, check out your new body awareness by answering the following simple questions. Groups, feel free to divide into teams and distribute paper and pens, and have a quizmaster to read them out aloud. The questions can also be downloaded and printed from www.nickhernbooks.co.uk/alexander-technique

The Quiz

1. The head weighs three, five or eight kilos?

2. The atlanto-occipital joint is where the skull meets the spine: true or false?

3. Is the greatest rotation of the spine at the lumbar, thoracic or cervical area?

4. Is the supporting area in the spine at the front or the back?

5. The spine meets the pelvis at the sacroiliac joint: true or false?

6. We sit better on a chair when using the pelvis or the coccyx?

7. If the first joints of the upper limb are in the fingers, where is the last joint?

8. If the fingers are the beginning of the upper limb, where is the end?

9. If you are six feet tall, what is your wingspan?

10. Do the collarbones sit higher or lower than the shoulder blades?

11. Is the shoulder joint at the back and side of the top of the upper arm, or somewhere near the front of the armpit?

12. How many bones are there in the foot?

13. Are the hip joints where the legs meet the pelvis in the groin area, or at the top of the pelvis?

14. The waist joint is between the ribs and the pelvis: true or false?

15. Do the lungs start above or below the collarbones?

16. The diaphragm is attached to the ribs, the tip of the breastbone and the _ P _ _ _ .

17. The ribs are jointed to the spine and hang downwards from there: true or false?

18. Does the heart rise or fall as we sing?

Look up the answers in Appendix D on page 283 – and award yourself eighteen out of eighteen!

Then and Now

Drawing Yourself Again

On a piece of A4 paper, draw a picture of yourself with your non-dominant hand whilst listening to baroque music and enjoying a sweetie. On the back of the paper, write what you feel you have achieved through this course – which habits have you addressed and, occasionally, managed to change? Which, of all the experiments and principles, did you find worked for you? When you have finished, find the original drawing and the comments you made at the beginning of the course and compare them to these later ones. Check out each other's drawings in a group – it is fun to see how other people's pictures have changed or not. This is not a psychological profile but it is interesting to note any shifts. I remember a student who arrived as quite a shy sort but found his confidence over the two years I was working with him. His first picture was drawn in pencil, except for piercing blue eyes. He still had those in his second picture, but this time the rest of him was coloured in too.

Go Compare

Look back at today's film and then at the one you made right at the beginning of the course. How do they compare? You now have them both as a record of your early progress. It has only been eleven weeks, so don't expect miracles – and yet, why not? Sometimes it does happen that giant leaps have already been made. It may just be the confidence you exude on camera, even if you see that you are still pulling your head back as you sit and stand, bracing your legs, stooping to pick something up, arching your back as you put something on a high shelf and rolling from side to side as you walk. We can get better at what we do, or we can change what we do. And maybe you are able to maintain a free, easy balance as you speak and sing and act.

And the Future...?

So now you ask, 'Where do I go from here? Is that it? When can I stop being aware of how I am doing things?' Once awakened, once 'online', we will never go completely 'offline' again – and, indeed, why would we want to return to a state of unconsciousness? But if we change our use, we create a new neural pathway or network, a new habit, and it will very quickly be brought to our attention if it needs changing again. And now we have the tools to do that. F. M. sums it up like this:

> '...once that control has been mastered, the actual movements that follow are given in charge of the subconscious self, although always on the understanding that a counter order may be given at any moment. Thus it will be seen that the difference between the new habit and the old is that the old was our master and ruled us, whilst the new is our servant ready to carry out our lightest wish without question though always working quietly and unobtrusively on our behalf in accordance with the most recent orders given.'[2]

The next step could be to find yourself an Alexander teacher and get some individual or small-group coaching online. This can be very effective, but if you can experience some 'hands-on' instruction as a supplement for your own continuing experiments, I do recommend this. The hands-on experience with an Alexander teacher is very special. Human beings are sensitive. When we shake someone's hand, we instantly get information from them: tentative, confident, hard, soft, awake, limp. As soon as we touch someone else, our balance affects and is affected by the other person. When you are in the presence of a teacher who has been playing intensely with this stuff for at least three years, and they put their hands on you and you receive their touch, you are going to fly! A teacher can sense if you are holding or freeing yourself up. Your system wants to be in an easy place, so if the teacher is in an open, free place, then you will come into rapport and find yourself opening to this new experience without having to do anything! You are dancing with each other, being sensitive to each other.

In the Appendices you will find contact details, so you can see if there is an Alexander wizard in your area. (We often live down the road from you muggles. In disguise. Waiting for you.) You can always continue to log your own experiments and discoveries. Keep your attention spatially active and present. Lie down! Do nothing! Think of something funny; whisper an 'ah'; step into cardboard boxes; clean your teeth in semiflexion; step onto a travelator; let your arms be wings; let your Higher Creative Self out to play; think from your magic lemon. Life can be a party! (Magic lemon? You mean I haven't given you your magic lemon? How did that happen? Ah well, as they say, always leave them wanting more...)

Good luck with the rest of your journey, and thank you for your attention and company so far. It's always an honour to accompany someone in their learning, even if I don't know that I am!

'Always keep Ithaca in your heart.
That is your final destination.
But don't rush the journey in the least.
It's better to make it last for years
And when you finally come to the island to rest, an
    aged one,
Wealthy with all that you have gained on the way
Do not expect Ithaca to give you any riches…
Ithaca gave you a beautiful journey.'[3]

(Okay, if you ever have a lesson with me, I promise I will give you a magic lemon…)

Acknowledgements

Thank you to:

Nick Hern and Matt Applewhite for giving me the space to learn how to write a book, their trust that I would come up with the goods, and for their astonishing expertise in commas.

Jenny Quick for the fabulous illustrations.

Toby O'Connor and Kim Plowright for technical help with recordings.

All my Alexander teachers along the way for their compassion, kindness, patience and humour, especially David Gorman who opened up my reasoning brain, Margaret Edis who gave me back my trust in the world and my hip joints, Tommy Thompson my heart, Rivka Cohen the earth, Ilana Machover my back, and to dear Maitreyi aka Judy Senior, who told me that one day I would write a book on this stuff. (How did you know?!) These few words cannot begin to express the influence you all had on my life and my deep gratitude.

All my Alexander colleagues for their encouragement and advice, including Judith Kleinman, Peter Nobes, Tim Cacciatore, Sue Laurie, Robin Simmons, Jean Fischer and MaryJean Allan, to Wolfgang Weisner for his wonderful work with peacock feathers and tightropes, Barbara Conable who introduced me to 'Fred' my 18" Johns Hopkins skeleton, and Jackie Beim for her beautifully out-of-tune rendition of 'Summertime' one sunset on Alonnisos.

All my drama students, friends and colleagues from Arts Educational Schools London, who taught me so much over the years and gave me such wonderful space and time to play in. What a collaboration we had!

All my other amazing students, friends and companions on this journey who cannot be categorised, including Robert Lewis, Nikita Roure, Adele Salem, Waltraud and Uschi for champagne, and at the Alfa Café on Alonnisos, Lee and Evangelia for encouraging me with bottomless cups of coffee and pastries as I scribbled away.

Very special thanks to Alexander teachers and friends Christos Noulis and Julia Messenger for going over the manuscript with their Alexander specs for anything too outrageous or untrue. To Christos a second time for his invaluable support, insights, practical advice and friendship throughout the whole process, always there at the end of an email/text/video call to cheer me on when my own 'up' direction was being a little elusive.

And last, but not least, here's to Mo, my darling husband for being himself, my rock.

Notes and References

Epigraph

1. 'Ithaca' by C. P. Cavafy, private translation by Pakis Athanasiou (edited by Penny O'Connor).

Introduction

1. Wilfred Barlow, *The Alexander Principle* (Orion, London, 2001 paperback ed.), p. 15.

Lesson One

1. F. M. Alexander, *Man's Supreme Inheritance* (Mouritz, London, 2002 ed.), p. 65.

2. Nancy Friday, *My Mother Myself* (HarperCollins, London, 1994 paperback ed.), pp. 417–8.

3. Channel 4 and Discovery Channel, *Body Story*, Episode 7: 'Out of Control', DigitalNetHD 2014, youtu.be/UWrGz9tIZjI

4. There are many sayings from Alexander handed down by teachers who worked with him, and I believe this to be one of them. It's a corruption of Oscar Wilde's 'Life is too important to be taken seriously.'

5. R. Gu, J. H. Zhou, Jihua Zhnang and Mei Song Tong, 'The baroque music's influence on learning efficiency based on the research of brain cognition': Conference paper, 35th Progress in Electromagnetics Research Symposium, China (Aug 2014). Published at www.researchgate.net

6. F. M. Alexander, 'Teaching Aphorisms' in *Articles and Lectures*, ed. Jean M. O. Fischer (Mouritz, London, 1995), p. 207.

7. Jonathan Pryce, *Guardian*: 'The Q & A' (7 March, 2015).

8. F. M. Alexander, 'Teaching Aphorisms', p. 197.

Lesson Two

1. Frank Pierce Jones, *Freedom to Change* (Mouritz, London, 1960), Appendix D, p. 192.

2. F. M. Alexander, *Man's Supreme Inheritance* (Mouritz, London, 2002 ed.), p. 64.

3. Nick Moseley, *Meisner in Practice* (Nick Hern Books, London, 2012).

4. Marion Milner, *A Life of One's Own* (Virago Press, London, 1986), p. 105.

5. Les Fehmi and Jim Robbins, *The Open-Focus Brain: Harnessing the Power of Attention to Heal Mind and Body* (Trumpeter Books, Boston, 2007).

6. W. H. Davies, 'Leisure', *Collected Poems* (Forgotten Books, London, 2012).

7. F. M. Alexander, *Man's Supreme Inheritance*, p 64.

8. D. T. Suzuki, 'Zen and Swordsmanship' in *Zen and Japanese Culture* (Princeton University Press, 2019), p. 107.

Lesson Three

1. See the 'Hawthorne effect' on Wikipedia: en.wikipedia.org/wiki/Hawthorne_effect

2. Richard Roche, Sean Commins (eds.), *Pioneering Studies in Cognitive Neuroscience* (McGraw-Hill Education, UK, 2009), pp. 22–55.

3. F. M. Alexander, *The Use of the Self* (Orion Spring, 2018) pp. 46–7.

4. Robert Frost, 'The Road Not Taken' from *The Road Not Taken and Other Poems*, ed. David Orr (Penguin/Random House, London, 2015 ed.).

5. F. M. Alexander, *The Universal Constant in Living* (Mouritz, 2000), p. 83.

6. Kathryn Caster, 'The Centipede's Dilemma' (1871): 'The Centipede was happy – quite! / Until a toad in fun / Said, "Pray, which leg goes after which?" / This raised her doubts to such a pitch / She fell exhausted in a ditch / Not knowing how to run.'

7. Sandra Blakeslee and Matthew Blakeslee, *The Body has a Mind of Its Own: How Body Maps in Your Brain Help You Do (Almost) Everything Better* (Random House, USA Inc, May 2009 paperback ed.).

8. There was a movement that began in late 1970s for Alexander teachers to be better informed regarding anatomy, to know what was where and how we functioned as a whole system. My trainer David Gorman wrote

and illustrated by hand the bible for Alexander teachers, *The Body Moveable* – available from Amazon or www.bodymoveable.com – and runs an online course on the Anatomy of Wholeness and a series of articles on Design and Function at www.learningmethods.com. Barbara Conable has written a number of books, including *What Every Musician Needs to Know About the Body* (Andover Press, USA, 1998), and is founder of Andover Educators, which trains and licenses music teachers to teach a six-hour Body Mapping course.

9. Robert Frost, 'The Silken Tent' from *The Poetry of Robert Frost.* (Holt (Henry) & Co, U.S., 1979, 1st Owl Books ed.).

10. F. M. Alexander, *The Universal Constant in Living,* p.116.

Lesson Four

1. youtu.be/oEA18Y8gM0, 'The World's Fastest Runner' (National Geographic, 8 May 2013).

2. I want to acknowledge the work of Moshe Feldenkrais. I learned these experiments with the eyes from my Feldenkrais teacher Scott Clark. Feldenkrais himself had Alexander lessons with renowned teacher Walter Carrington whilst Alexander was still alive. When Alexander heard Feldenkrais was in the building he asked him to leave as he thought he was stealing his ideas. Imagine if, instead, they had become collaborators!

3. Rollo May, *The Courage to Create* (Norton, New York and London, 1975) p. 130.

Lesson Five

1. Marion Milner, *A Life of One's Own* (Virago, London, 1986), p. 102.

2. F. M. Alexander, *The Universal Constant in Living* (Mouritz, 2000), pp. 87–8.

3. I recommend *Lessons from the Art of Juggling: How to Achieve Your Full Potential in Business Learning and Life* by Michael Gelb (inspirational speaker and Alexander teacher) and Tony Buzan (Harmony, 1994).

4. Daniel Goleman, 'Lesson: The Universality of Emotion, Subsection: Between Impulse and Action: Leverage Points in the Mind' in *Destructive Emotions* (Bloomsbury, London, 2004), pp. 144–50.

5. Phillip V. Tobias, *Man: The Tottering Biped: The Evolution of His Posture, Poise and Skill*

6 Ian McEwan, *Atonement* (Vintage, London, 2002 ed.), p. 35.

Lesson Six

1. From Rilke's poem 'How Surely Gravity's Law' from *The Book of Hours*, translated by Anita Barrows and Joanna Macy (Riverhead Books, 2005).

2. Phillip V. Tobias, *Man: The Tottering Biped: The Evolution of His Posture, Poise and Skill* (UNSWP: University of New South Wales Press/Committee in Postgraduate Medical Education, Sydney, 1982). Although Tobias used the term 'tottering biped' in the title of his book, he acknowledges that it was originally coined by Earnest Albert Hooton, a physical anthropologist at Harvard University.

3. Oliver Sacks, *The Man Who Mistook His Wife for a Hat* (Duckworth, London, 1985).

4. From Rilke's poem 'How Surely Gravity's Law'.

5. Professor Eyal Lederman, *The Myth of Core Stability*: www.cpdo.net/Lederman_The_myth_of_core_stability.pdf in CPDO Online Journal (June 2007), p. 1–17. www.cpdo.net, section 'The Strength Issue', p. 5.

6. William Shakespeare, *Romeo and Juliet*, Act Two, Scene One.

Lesson Seven

1. T. S. Eliot, 'Burnt Norton' in *Four Quartets* (Faber and Faber, London, 1944).

2. 'In our uprightness we are probably the most precarious of all the creatures with so much of our body so high up over so many free joints. Precisely because we are so much up over ourselves, we also have the possibility of being one of the most balanced of creatures (albeit a possibility more often than not unrealised). In fact, it is this very instability in our balance that enables us to effectively use the potential energy of our height. At the same time it is the balance in our instability that allows us such a potentially low overhead in terms of energy expended in staying upright.' David Gorman, Part 3. 'From the Ground Up' in *In Our Own Image*, eight-part series on Human Design and Function, www.learningmethods.com/image3.htm, reprinted from *The Alexander Review*, Vol. 1, No. 3, Sept 1986.

3. Robert Browning, 'Andrea del Sarto' (also called 'The Faultless Painter', 1855), but often associated with architect Ludwig Mies van der Rohe, who used the phrase in 1947 as a precept for minimalist design.

4. A. A. Milne, 'Halfway Down' in *When We Were Very Young* (Egmont, 2016, first published 1924).

5. There are a number of other exercises you can find on the internet. The two I favour were given to me by Scott Clark, Feldenkrais teacher. As

with all activities, it is possible to use Alexander awareness, inhibition and direction to do them well. Lying on the floor, hold one knee to your chest as you lengthen the other one out, keeping it raised off the floor. The knee raised to the chest is stopping the arching and the straight leg is stretching the psoas. Swap legs. In the other exercise, lie on your back in semi-supine, raise the feet a few inches up from the floor and then let both knees go to the side and do tiny scissor movements up and down. Just ten, maybe, then rest in semi-supine, then ten to the other side.

6. Andrew Shields and Malcom Balk, *The Art of Running: Raising Your Performance with the Alexander Technique* (Collins & Brown, 2016).

7. F. M. Alexander, 'Teaching Aphorisms' in *Articles and Lectures* (Mouritz, 1995), p. 194.

8. William Shakespeare, *Hamlet*, Act Three, Scene Two.

Lesson Eight

1. F. M. Alexander, *Aphorisms*, ed. Jean M. O. Fischer (Mouritz, 2000), p. 60.

2. David Gorman, *Looking at Ourselves: Articles, Lectures and Columns 1984–1996* (Learning Methods, 1997), p. 60.

3. Phrase taken from title of Janet Feindel's *The Thought Propels the Sound* (Plural Publishing Inc, 2008).

4. youtu.be/hp-gCvW8PRY, '3D Yoga – View of diaphragm during respiration'.

5. youtu.be/apFui6-ffnM; the full animation of The Art of Breathing can be found at jessicawolfartofbreathing.com.

6. David Gorman, *Looking at Ourselves*, p. 27.

7. F. M. Alexander, *Aphorisms*, p. 38.

8. youtu.be/p-cW4a8i5_E, 'Normal TMJ Function', Edith Gardener, 29 July 2014.

9. F. M. Alexander, *Aphorisms*, p. 84.

10. William Blake, 'Eternity' (1880).

Lesson Nine

1. Sheila Peltz Weinberg, 'Untie' (shlomohsherman.com/literary/poems/fanpoems/weinberg.html).

2. 'Summertime' from *Porgy and Bess* (1935) by George and Ira Gershwin.

3. The flipper movement is usually made with the palm of the hand down, but I have found that whilst in semi-supine having the palm up keeps the

chest open more easily by not pulling the shoulder in – very useful for those with habitually pulled-in shoulders. You can read more about the Dart Procedures in Robin Simmons' book *The Evolution of Movement: A Guide to the Procedures Originated by Raymond Dart* (Mouritz, 2018, second revised ed.).

4. F. M. Alexander, *Aphorisms*, p. 72.

5. *Ibid*, endpaper.

Lesson Ten

1. W. B. Yeats, 'A Prayer for Old Age', first published in *The Spectator*, 1934.

2. F. M. Alexander, *Aphorisms*, p. 88.

3. Thanks to Lee Warren, Alexander colleague, magician and inspirational speaker, who worked with me as an assistant at ArtsEd, and whose inspiring work I developed into this exercise.

4. I recommend *To the Actor: On the Technique of Acting* by Michael Chekhov, presently published by Martino Fine Books, 2014.

5. Metaphor taken from lecture by David Gorman at the Centre for Training, *c*.1991.

6. Nick Moseley, *Meisner in Practice* (Nick Hern Books, London, 2012).

7. William Shakespeare, *Hamlet*, Act Five, Scene Two.

8. Michael J. Gelb, *Present Yourself* (Jalmar Press, 1988).

9. William Shakespeare, *Hamlet*, Act Two, Scene Two.

10. F. M. Alexander, *Aphorisms*, p. 23.

Lesson Eleven

1. Joseph Campbell and Bill Moyers, *The Power of Myth* (Anchor, 1988), p. 4.

2. F. M. Alexander, *Man's Supreme Inheritance* (Mouritz, 2002), p. 55.

3. 'Ithaca' by C. P. Kavafy, private translation by Pakis Athanasiou (and edited by Penny O'Connor).

Appendices

Appendix A

Audio Script for Lying in Semi-supine

As you lie there in semi-supine – head supported, knees bent and the feet spreading onto the floor – without you having to do anything, the neck is freeing, the head is being released away from the spine, the whole back is lengthening and widening, the limbs are lengthening and releasing out of their habitual tensions, the knees are easily balancing up and the feet spreading onto the floor... And as you lie there, take in what's around you. See what you see. Notice not just the ceiling but what's in your peripheral vision... Allow yourself to tune in to what you can hear, the sounds around... and become of aware of what you are in touch with: the ground under your back supporting you, the air on your skin, your clothes... Perhaps you can sense the fragrance of the space you are lying in, the taste in your mouth... All this, that you take in all the time *un*consciously, you are now taking in consciously... And as you allow yourself to become more present – taking in the world around you, seeing what you see, hearing what you hear, sensing what you sense – the neck continues to free itself and the head continues to release from the spine, the spine lengthening as it obeys the laws of gravity, and any excessive curves gently lessening. The shoulders are widening away from each other; the pelvis releasing; the hip, knee and ankle joints freeing up and the feet spreading onto the floor... As you lie there witnessing yourself and the world but not doing anything, it may be possible for you to become aware of the distance between yourself and the ceiling, the space that's there... Perhaps it's possible also to note the distance between the top of your head and the wall behind you, and the space that's there; the end of your feet and the wall beyond your feet, the space that's there; the distance between the left side of you and the wall to the left; the right side of you and the wall to your right and the space that's there... and noticing all these parameters of space one after the other, all at the same time... the floor beneath you, supporting you, coming up to meet you.

And as you lie there, let me take you on a journey through the internal space that also exists; the space that you take up, right here, right now... We usually pay attention to the matter that we can see, but we know that the ratio of space between the atomic particles is equivalent to the distance between the earth and the moon, for example. So let us pay attention to all that space that exists within us. Consider the distance between the top of your head and the roof of your mouth; between the front of your eyes and the back of your head; between your right ear and your left ear... It may now be possible for you to have a sense of the whole volume of space that is your head...

Be aware of the distance between the front of your lips and the back of your throat; between the roof of your mouth and the top of your larynx; between the inside of your left cheek and the inside of your right cheek, so you have a sense of the whole volume of space that is your mouth. And add that to the volume of space that is your head...

And thinking of that place just behind your ear, between the skull and the jaw, maybe you can think of the distance between the top of your neck there and the top of your ribs, the length of your neck; the distance between the left side of your neck and the right side of your neck, the left shoulder joint and the right shoulder joint; the distance between the front of the collarbones and the back of the shoulder blades; between the front of your throat and the back of your neck, so you have a sense of the whole volume of space that is your neck and shoulders. Add this to the volume of space that is your mouth and head...

And thinking of the distance between the shoulder joints and the elbows, the elbows and the wrists, the wrists and the tips of your fingers; the distance between the thumb and the little finger, the corresponding sides of the arm; the palm of the hand and the back of the hand; the inside of the arm and the back of the arm... Maybe it's possible to have a sense of the whole volume of space that is your arms, and add that to the volume of space that is your shoulders, neck, mouth and head...

And as you lie there, perhaps you can imagine the distance between the top of your ribs and the sitting bones, the bottom of your pelvis; and the distance between the left side of your torso, and the right side of your torso; the distance between the breastbone and the back of your spine, your belly and the back of your spine... So it may now be possible to have a sense of the whole volume of space that is your torso, noticing as you do how that volume of space changes as you allow the air to enter and exit either through your nose or your mouth.

And you can spend some time noting that portal between the outside world and the inside world, where the air enters and exits. Perhaps it comes in through the nose and out through the mouth; perhaps you can feel which nostril is engaged and when it changes. It doesn't really matter which gateway you use, as the air enters and exits all on its own, everything moving easily to allow this to happen, allowing the volume of space of your torso, the shape of your torso to change. Add that sense of the volume of space of your torso to the volume of space that is your arms and shoulders, neck, mouth and head...

And now we come to the legs. Perhaps it is possible for you to think of the distance between your hip joints and your knees, your knees and your ankles, your ankles and the soles of your feet. Give a thought also to the distance between the outside and the inside of your legs, the outside and the inside of your feet; the distance between the toes and the heels, and the distance between the front and the back of your legs. Now you may be able to sense the whole volume of space that is your legs, and add this to the volume of space that is your torso, your arms, your shoulders, neck, mouth and head…

So now, lying here, you have a sense of the whole volume of space that is you, from the top of your head to the soles of your feet, in the space that is around you.

If your eyes have closed, allow them to open gently and take in what is around you. Allow the light to fall into your eye. Perhaps you can hear other sounds beyond this voice through your earphones? Be aware of the floor beneath you: does it seem that there is more of you on the floor? Has something changed in you since you first lay down? Whatever you sense, whatever your experience, it is entirely valid. This is your journey and your discovery.

In a moment I am going to suggest that you come to standing, but let's go over it in your imagination first. And I want you to imagine coming to standing really easily and effortlessly. Imagine yourself letting your eyes drop to one side, the head following the eyes, and the opposing arm dropping over to begin an easy rotation through your whole body so that you find yourself supported on all-fours. This is an easy, flowing, speedy movement, the legs remaining bent as you use the momentum to curl over onto all fours. In your imagination you are allowing the spine to lengthen all the way to your ears; your eyes looking at the floor, the top of your head directed towards the opposing wall. There is slightly more support on the knees than the hands. And in your imagination you are allowing yourself to rock forward and back a little way before dropping back onto your heels. You are looking forward now, rocking back up to high kneeling, bringing one foot forward and imagining your head leading you up to full standing. It's so easy and effortless and flowing, it's almost as though you are floating up. And in your imagination – as you stand there for a few moments, thinking of the space above, behind and on either side, having a panoramic vision of what is in front of you, finding the weight more on the back of the foot – you can allow yourself to walk effortlessly away, keeping these spatial directions in your mind as you go about your daily routines.

Now, having imagined this easy way of getting up, have a go. Come to full standing, rolling over into the future you just created for yourself.

Appendix B

Here are the lungs, trachea and diaphragm

See page 192.

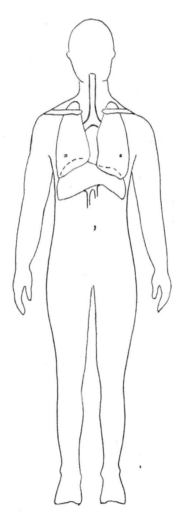

Appendix C

The Moon Like a Bone in the Sky: A Happening

The following instructions are for twelve people but the piece can be adapted for five or fewer. The first five instructions are the most important. I suggest you download and print the resource sheet from www.nickhernbooks.co.uk/alexander-technique, or photocopy the instructions, cut them up and dish out one instruction per person. It is like receiving a secret message! It is more exciting and in the moment if the actors don't compare notes or know who else is saying what or when. This exercise takes five minutes.

1. Stand in the centre of the space, looking at the clock or your watch. Look occasionally at the action going on around you. Call out the minutes, one to five, as the time goes by.

2. Sit on a chair looking at the sky. Every time the minutes are called out, stand up and point to the sky and exclaim: 'The Moon!' Hear the response: 'Like a bone in the sky', and look to and reply to that person: 'You're shivering'. When someone stops sobbing, sit down again. Repeat until the five minutes is called. Do as before but this time, when someone stops sobbing, keep standing instead of sitting.

3. Lie down. Whenever you hear the line 'You're shivering', wait for a beat, then turn over into a foetal shape and sob so that all can hear for a count of five. Then stop and turn back.

4. Stand shivering, occasionally rubbing your arms, waiting for someone to find you. Sometimes you can hum. Every time you hear the minutes called out, stop. When someone says: 'The Moon', look up at the sky with wonder. Wait until someone stops sobbing, then move to another space and continue shivering. Repeat until the five minutes is called. Then stop and, when someone says: 'The Moon', keep looking up at the sky with wonder.

5. Place a chair and sit on it, looking slightly down at the floor. Every time you hear the minutes called out, look up. When someone says: 'The Moon', run to them, look where they are pointing and exclaim with wonder: 'Like a bone in the sky.' After their response, turn and kiss them on the forehead. When someone stops sobbing, run back and sit down as before. Repeat until the five minutes is called. Then as before, but instead of running back to your chair, stay where you are.

6. Skip five steps. Stop: consider. Skip another five steps, perhaps in a different direction. From time to time you can sing 'Girls and Boys Come Out to Play' quietly. Every time you hear the minutes called out, stop. When someone says: 'The Moon', look up at the sky with wonder. Wait until someone stops sobbing, then continue as before. Repeat until the five minutes is called. Then stop and when someone says: 'The Moon', keep looking up at the sky with wonder.

7. Choose someone to look at with malice. Every time you hear the minutes called out, stop. When someone says: 'The Moon', look up at the sky with wonder. Wait until

someone stops sobbing, then move to another space and choose another person to look at maliciously. Repeat until the five minutes is called. Then stop and, when someone says: 'The Moon', keep looking up at the sky with wonder.

8. Choose someone to shadow, thinking of how much you love them. Every time you hear the minutes called out, stop. When someone says: 'The Moon', look up at the sky with wonder. Wait until someone stops sobbing, then choose a different person to shadow. Repeat until the five minutes is called. Then stop and when someone says: 'The Moon', keep looking up at the sky with wonder.

9. Walk slowly round the perimeter of the space, taking everything in. Every time you hear the minutes called out, stop. When someone says: 'The Moon', look up at the sky with wonder. Wait until someone finishes sobbing, then continue walking but round the other way. Repeat until the five minutes is called. Then stop and, when someone says: 'The Moon', keep looking up at the sky with wonder.

10. Notice someone walking round the perimeter of the space. Walk the perimeter too, but in the opposite direction, head down. But when you pass each other, touch her/his arm and look longingly after her/him for a moment before returning to your own walking. Every time you hear the minutes called out, stop. When someone says: 'The Moon', look up at the sky with wonder. Wait until someone finishes sobbing, then continue walking but round the other way. Repeat until the five minutes is called. Then stop and, when someone says: 'The Moon', keep looking up at the sky with wonder.

11. Kneel on the floor. Slowly turn your head from side to side. Five times in the whole piece randomly make a high-pitched 'oooo' sound, lasting five seconds. Every time you hear the minutes called out, stop turning your head or

making a sound. When someone says: 'The Moon', look up at the sky with wonder. Wait until someone stops sobbing, then move to another space and continue. Repeat until the five minutes is called. Then stop and when someone says: 'The Moon', keep looking up at the sky with wonder.

12. During the five minutes, whisper in the ear of each person: 'I love you.' Only once to each person. When someone says: 'The Moon', look up at the sky with wonder. Wait until someone stops sobbing, then move again. Stop when the five minutes is called and, when someone says: 'The Moon', keep looking up at the sky with wonder.

Appendix D

Answers to the Quiz

See page 257.

1. The head weighs about five kilos or ten pounds.

2. True: the atlanto-occipital joint is where the skull meets the spine.

3. The greatest rotation of the spine is at the cervical (neck) area.

4. The supporting area of the spine is at the front. Spinal processes at the back are for muscle and rib attachment, and a channel for the spinal cord.

5. True: the spine meets the pelvis at the sacroiliac joint.

6. We sit better on a chair when using the pelvis. The bottom of the pelvis is called 'the sitting bones'! If we sit on the coccyx, we are compressing the spine.

7. The last joint is the sternoclavicular, but you can say 'where the collarbone meets the breastbone.'

8. The end is perhaps where the latissimus dorsi meets the crest of the pelvis.

9. If you are six foot tall, your wing span is six foot.

10. The collarbones sit higher than the shoulder blades.

11. The shoulder joint is at the back and side at the top of our upper arm.

12. There are twenty-six bones in the foot.

13. The hip joints are where the legs meet the pelvis in the groin area.

14. Fake news: we don't have a waist joint!

15. The lungs start above the collarbones.

16. The diaphragm is attached to the ribs, the tip of the breastbone and the SPINE.

17. True: from the back the ribs drop downwards from the spine. Like Christmas-tree branches.

18. The heart rises as we sing. It sits on the diaphragm and the dome of the diaphragm rises as we breathe out.

Appendix E

The Alexander Principles

These are the Alexander Principles as I perceive them in this moment. Our understanding changes as we continue to practise.

Experiment
To discover how you do things and find ways of changing them.

Use Affects Function
Our habits affect how well we carry out activities.

Primary Control
The relationship of the head–neck–back which governs the rest of us.

Inhibition
Stopping our immediate reaction to a stimulus, momentarily giving up our intention. In the moment we create a gap between a stimulus and our habitual response, we can stop messages from the brain travelling down the old neural pathways and give ourselves other options.

Direction

A conscious instruction or order from the brain to the body, allowing the thought to reorganise us; and the direction we move in space: e.g. when we stop pulling ourselves down, we go in an 'up' direction.

Alexander's Directions or Orders

I'm allowing my neck to be free so that my head goes forward and up, so that my back lengthens and widens, and my knees go forward and away. (Instructions to give to ourselves 'one after the other, all at the same time'.) Directing the head to go forward and up can be awkward to consider. I have sometimes changed that in the text to the head rising. If Alexander was pulling his head back and down into his spine, he wanted it to go forward and up instead.

Conscious Awareness

An awareness of how we use ourselves; a unified field of attention that takes in the self, the world around us and our activity. The cultivation of being 'present in the moment'.

Faulty Sensory Appreciation

That we may not be doing what we think we're doing, and what seems right may be wrong and what seems wrong may be right.

End-gaining

Narrowing our attention too much to the end result, so that we are not able to give sufficient attention to the 'process' or how we are doing things. In order to change, we need to inhibit our end-gaining and live more in the present moment.

Psychophysical Unity

We are whole, not a divided self of mind and body – what affects one part of the system, affects the whole.

Non-doing

Allowing things to happen easily, rather than trying hard to get things right.

Spatial Directions

Think of the space above, behind and on either side, with a widened vision of the space in front, and sense the ground beneath your feet. One after the other, all at the same time. Please note these are not part of the original directions Alexander gave himself, but I give them here as a reminder to help you find the dynamic relationship of the head, neck and back, and come into a unified field of attention.

Appendix F

Some Alexander Organisations and Websites

The following websites have useful information on Alexander Technique, including the major Alexander societies in the world and their lists of teachers, as well as information on the work:

Society of Teachers of the Alexander Technique (STAT), UK:
www.alexandertechnique.co.uk

The International Affiliated Societies of STAT:
www.alexandertechniqueworldwide.org

International body of teachers not affiliated to STAT:
www.alexandertechniqueinternational.com

Information on Alexander Technique:
www.alexandertechnique.com

Penny's website:
www.alexanderpen.co.uk

List of Exercises

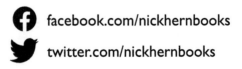